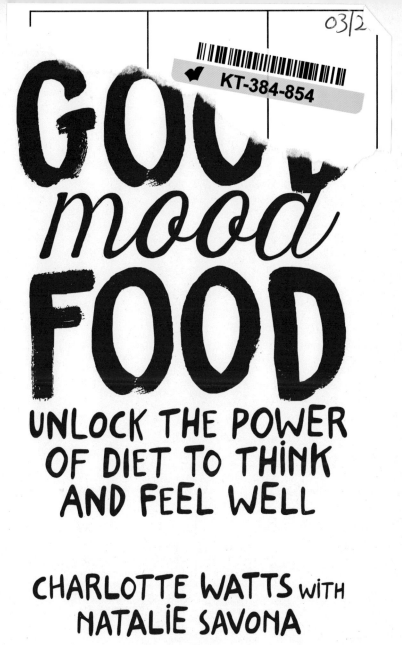

GOOD mood FOOD

UNLOCK THE POWER OF DIET TO THINK AND FEEL WELL

CHARLOTTE WATTS with NATALIE SAVONA

This edition published in the UK and USA 2018 by
Nourish, an imprint of Watkins Media Limited
89–93 Shepperton Road
London N1 3DF

enquiries@nourishbooks.com

Design and typography copyright © Watkins Media Limited 2018
Text Copyright © Charlotte Watts and Natalie Savona

1 3 5 7 9 10 8 6 4 2

Commissioning Editor: Kate Fox
Managing Editor: Daniel Hurst
Editor: Helena Caldon
Head of Design: Georgina Hewitt
Typeset by: seagulls.net
Production: Uzma Taj

Printed and bound in Great Britain by TJ International

A CIP record for this book is available from the British Library

ISBN: 978-1-84899-360-0

www.watkinspublishing.com

Note/Disclaimer: The material contained in this book is set out in good faith for general
guidance and no liability can be accepted for loss or expense incurred in relying on
the information given. In particular this book is not intended to replace expert medical
or psychiatric advice. This book is for informational purposes only and is for your own
personal use and guidance. It is not intended to diagnose, treat, or act as a substitute for
professional medical advice. The author is not a medical practitioner nor a counsellor, and
professional advice should be sought if desired before embarking on any health-related
programme.

A note on the authors: The recipes in this book have previously been published
in *The Kitchen Shrink* by Natalie Savona. The remainder of the text, while influenced
by *The Kitchen Shrink*, is an original work by Charlotte Watts and should be accredited
to her.

CONTENTS

INTRODUCTION

Welcome to this book, which I've designed to support your good mood, but also along the way I hope it will inspire an interest in nutritious and delicious food. Understanding how what we eat changes how we feel, can help us tune into the very real effects of nutrition, and so motivate us to make the best choices. Mood disorders are now affecting more of us than ever before, but through exploration of the nutritional factors that contribute to them, we are able to see practical, realistic and sustainable antidotes to conditions that interfere with our quality of life.

Natalie Savona, author of *The Kitchen Shrink*, and I studied and tutored at the same college (the Institute for Optimum Nutrition, London) and we have similar outlooks for nutrition, believing that it is most importantly about enjoying food and tuning into our individual needs and that this approach can only support mood if we respond deeply to a sense of self-care and awareness. Although Natalie has moved on from nutrition now, I was delighted to be able to pick up her mantel and create a new work for this new time, using the content of her excellent book. Since the publication of Natalie's book in 2010, we have begun to understand even more of the mechanisms and links between the ways we eat, live, respond and our mental outlook, so *Good Mood Food* features more up-to-date information.

Conditions that affect your mood, mind and energy come in many forms and even more degrees of seriousness. It may be that you feel persistently low; you may find that you are often irritable or turning to food for a boost; you may suffer from premenstrual syndrome or seasonal affective disorder; you may have difficulty sleeping or perhaps you are finding that your brain power is not what it used to be. One thing that all these various problems have in common is that they are inextricably linked to your diet. Throughout this book, we will help you to sustain a more buoyant mood by examining in detail a number of the more common mood-related conditions, such as insomnia and cravings, and exploring how to overcome them using nutritional methods.

We have all felt low at some time or another – it is absolutely normal to feel sad following a bereavement, at the end of a relationship, the loss of a job, a disappointment or a severe illness. However, for some people this sense of sadness goes on for months on end and permeates every aspect of their lives, leaving them unable to truly enjoy anything they do. They can even suffer from physical symptoms, such as fatigue, sleep problems and a change in appetite. Sometimes the sadness does not even have an obvious trigger, it just comes from nowhere in particular and lingers. Such a persistent mood disturbance may continue as mild depression for years, or in some cases it may be so severe that the sufferer is barely able to cope with normal daily life. This problem is more common than you might think – as much as one-fifth of the adult population in Europe and North America are thought to suffer from some degree of depression.

Mood disorders are notoriously difficult to categorize and deal with using conventional medical approaches, because they can be triggered by countless different sources. It is clear that the physical and psychological aspects of conditions such as depression and anxiety are closely linked. Major life events have an impact on our physical health, which in turn may affect our emotions, particularly in the long term, and so it is clear that any approach to redressing mood imbalances must take into account both the physical and psychological aspects. In reality, these are not two separate 'things', because every emotion we feel ripples through our body, and physical experience always involves the mind, too. To reiterate this point in this book, we use the term 'mind-body'.

Although the primary focus of this book is physiological strategies based on food, you will also find advice on how you can talk through problems (see pages 281-2). Anyone suffering from conditions such as severe depression should visit their doctor for a full medical evaluation, to ensure that any other treatment – be it drugs or psychotherapy – can be supported and can fully work with your nutritional strategies too. Adhering to the basic principles of healthy eating can make the healthiest of people feel even better, too. It follows that if you provide your body with good-quality 'fuel' and minimize your intake of substances that silt up your system, both your body and mind will work more efficiently for you. Much research has shown that diet and food supplements can relieve or even eliminate symptoms of all kinds of illnesses, not least those affecting the way our minds work.

Clearly, a diet that is rich in nutrients can improve your brain function and help you to combat low moods, but how can you ensure that your intake of nutrients is adequate? One school of thought is that if you have a balanced diet you are getting all the nutrients you need. However, it is important to remember that a great many of us do not actually eat this mythical (and often confusing) idea of a 'balanced diet' or understand what it might actually be. When many people under stress and time pressures are grabbing a sugary muffin for breakfast, nibble biscuits mid-morning, have a sandwich for lunch and then eat a ready-made meal in the evening, there is plenty of room for awareness. Even if our diet is not that bad, too few of us eat a varied diet of fresh, unprocessed, nutrient-rich foods most of the time. With our time pulled away by screens and ever-increasing amounts of information, redirecting this attention towards how we look after and nourish ourselves can have a truly great effect on our quality of life.

Knowing some basic requirements can help to guide you. Most governments have set recommended daily amounts of vitamins that each of us require, based on our sex and age. But the truth is that nobody knows exactly how much each of us needs, especially given our individual lifestyles, exercise routines and environments. We do know that our ancestors would have eaten different types of food on different days and throughout the changing seasons, and that their calorie intake would have varied greatly day to day, so that the idea of set mealtimes for each day doesn't follow the variations that our biology and metabolisms now expect. Our ancestors would have also had nutrient-dense food with none of the sugar and processed or junk food that we eat.

The government nutrient recommendations are probably conservative estimates and are generally aimed at the minimum amounts of micro-nutrients required to prevent the symptoms of deficiencies, rather than to optimize health. Worryingly, research worldwide has shown that significant numbers of men, women and children are currently not even getting these minimum recommended daily amounts of nutrients. For example, one survey in the UK found that 72 per cent of women and 42 per cent of men did not have an adequate intake of magnesium (this 'calming mineral' is discussed much in this book). As for the macro-nutrients – protein, fats and carbohydrates – most people in developed countries do get enough of these from their diet. That said, the form in which macro-nutrients are commonly consumed is often not healthy. Many people tend to eat refined flour in bread, high-fat animal protein and excess animal fats or fats that have been processed; many of the micro-nutrients contained in these foods have been lost during processing.

We are also exposed to many anti-nutrients – substances that deplete our stock of nutrients when they are processed in our bodies and that can add to stress on the mind-body and throw regulation of neurotransmitters (brain chemicals) and hormones out of whack. Fizzy drinks, sugar, coffee, tea, alcohol and cigarettes interfere with our body's ability to absorb minerals, as well as keeping us in cycles of craving the 'highs' of these stimulants and leaving us at the whim of a rollercoaster ride of mood and energy. So much of what we explore in this book isn't simply what is 'good' or 'bad'; not what we *should* or *shouldn't* be eating, but why we might crave these substances, how they relate to what we need and how we can unravel the cycles that keep us revisiting habits we would like to move past.

The first two chapters discuss the two most important, basic, underlying causes of mood issues in the twenty-first century: blood sugar imbalance and stress – these affect us all simply because of the way we tend to live in modern times, so here we will show you how to create the foundations to which you can add other factors. From there, in Chapters 3 and 4, we move on to supporting how we create and maintain balanced mental function, with some deeper nutritional specifics. Chapter 5 delves into the world of the gut and the liver; even if you do not have digestive issues, it is worth reading about how to support these areas as they are so fundamental for everybody's mental health. Chapter 6 addresses appetite regulation, which is especially useful if your efforts to effect sustainable change get rail-roaded by cravings and compulsive eating, but also helpful to understand the link between our mood and appetite drives. Chapter 7 is all about sleep quality; like digestion, you don't need to have 'problems' here to attend to this most important aspect of mood regulation – it's all about quality! Chapter 8 explains the relationship between female hormones and our mental states, including how this changes in our different phases, and there's some information here for men, too.

At the beginning of each section you will find checklists that are designed to give you a general indication of how issues in the area being discussed can show up. Remember, some of these can be signs of an underlying disease and the suggestions in the chapters are not intended to combat extreme states of illnesses. It is always advisable to check with your doctor before embarking on any health programme, especially if it involves significant changes to your usual diet. Similarly, if you are on medication do check with your physician about making radical changes to your diet or taking any nutritional supplements.

In Chapter 9 we put all this information and advice together with an overview of how to eat for good mood, and here we have put together a 7-day and a 14-day cleansing programme that you can follow –just choose whichever one you prefer to do or which best fits your situation.

Within the first eight chapters you will find a variety of recipes that don't just tell you what to eat but also help to tell the story of how specific ingredients, their nutrients and certain combinations can support your mental health. This is backed up with information to give you an understanding of the therapeutic qualities of food, and how you can play around with and explore the tastes and effects of different ingredients to create a diet that works best for you. Although the recipes are chosen for each chapter based on their relevance to the particular focuses being discussed, you'll get a feel for which ones are also beneficial and can be combined with other foods for optimal mental function. For instance, a recipe in Chapter 1 might feature protein for balancing blood sugar, which could mean that other protein-rich recipes in other chapters can help in that area, too. Nutrition is not as simplistic as one ingredient or combination of factors having an effect only in one part of the body; all parts of us are interconnected, so any positive change that you make in one area will ripple through all body systems.

Far from being merely essential fuel, food can also be a source of great pleasure and emotional comfort. Beyond simply satisfying our basic nutritional needs for brain function and nervous system regulation, our relationship with food can be a wonderful sensory journey where we discover that what nourishes us can also provide joy. When these two elements come together, we can relax into our personal food rhythm and really feel and understand what we need and when we need it. Then we don't have to feel the pressure to be perfect (or neurotic, as perfect really doesn't exist!) and we can instead enjoy the odd treat or diversion without self-criticism, and knowing how we can guide ourselves to get back on track to good mood food.

If the advice given here provokes more personal questions or you are confused about what suits you, consult a qualified nutritional therapist. They will also be able to recommend laboratory tests to help uncover underlying causes for any health concerns you have, if they think that is relevant.

I came to nutrition from my own personal health issues – including mental health, digestive and sleep issues – and this journey of working out how to help myself live with calm, symptom-free, was illuminating. My personal experiences and those of my clients are dotted through these pages, and I sincerely hope our stories are of help to you and open up as rewarding a journey for you!

Wishing you good mood
Charlotte

Part One
RECIPES TO GET YOU GOING

CHAPTER I

ENERGY AND BRAIN FUEL

We all know that when we feel happy and buoyant, life seems to take less effort and flow more easily, but when we get low, things can seem so very hard and easily drain us of energy that appears to be in rather short supply.

So we begin this book with the foundation of regulating mood, as well as energy and sleep: blood sugar balance. Nutritionally, this is the cornerstone of all the other considerations that we will explore in further chapters; when energy to our cells and brain is not consistent, all aspects of mental and physical health can be affected. An understanding of the systems in play and how we derive energy from the food we eat – and how it can so profoundly affect mood – can help us make changes that we feel make sense to improve mood. As our body responds to food that helps us find balance, we can access our own self-soothing abilities, feel calmer and find liberation from cycles of craving.

Recognizing our health patterns and behaviours provides clues to where the balance of energy supply may be disrupted. If you suffer from recurrent dives in mood, concentration and energy, or find that you often reach for a sugary snack or a cup of coffee to 'pick you up', only to find you feel grumpy and exhausted again shortly afterwards, blood sugar imbalance may be the culprit.

On the list below, tick the symptoms that apply to you regularly:

- Fatigue.
- Irritability.
- Cravings for sweet foods or drinks/coffee/tea/cigarettes.
- A need for regular snacks.
- Lapses in mood/concentration/memory.
- Difficulty making decisions.
- Light-headedness.
- Irritation or intolerance.
- 'Butterflies' in stomach for no apparent reason.
- Difficulty getting to sleep, or waking in the night.
- Headaches.
- Palpitations.

If you ticked six or more of the above symptoms, you may be having difficulty keeping your blood sugar balanced, in which case you are probably familiar with the following scenario. At around three o'clock in the afternoon, you suddenly start to yawn, then your concentration goes, and a black cloud seems to move over the day. But never mind, you know how to cure all that – a cup of coffee, a cigarette or a bar of chocolate soon does the trick, and you can get back to the task in hand . . . until the next slump strikes. This is when we feel disoriented by this bumpy journey through life.

Why do I feel this way?

Each one of our cells relies on a steady supply of glucose, the form of sugar we mainly use for energy (although we can use fats and proteins, too). When glucose that has been broken down from the carbohydrates in our food enters the bloodstream, the hormone insulin is released from the pancreas to move it into cells. Our brain demands much of this fuel as the human brain expends high levels of energy.

When these blood sugar levels become too low, the pancreas releases another hormone, glucagon, signals the release of stored sugar (as glycogen) from the liver and muscle to be broken down and released into the bloodstream. This should create a fairly constant level of sugar in the blood for continual and sustained body and brain energy throughout the day. Unfortunately, we tend to eat sugar in excess, beyond our fuel needs, in our modern diet and so our pancreas glands are called on to work hard to deal with more pronounced blood sugar 'highs and lows'.

What's the link with my diet?

Of course, you don't need us to tell you that what we eat affects our energy levels and that sometimes we make the wrong choices. Blood sugar levels that 'rollercoaster' outside of more consistent levels (see the chart on page 15) are what bring these highs and lows, and these in turn are linked to the food we eat and drink, offset in particular by eating sweet, sugary and starchy foods such as grains, beans and potatoes in large quantities. We know that such foods may temporarily fulfill a craving brought on by sudden tiredness and irritability, but they also cause our blood sugar levels – and with them our energy and mood – to rise quickly (the 'high'), then drop suddenly (the 'low' or crash). Maintaining even blood sugar levels is, therefore, one of the most crucial factors in supporting mental health stability, and every other issue that we have with moods that we discuss in the next few chapters builds on this.

Our bodies are very carefully designed to maintain balance (otherwise known as homoeostasis); for example, ensuring that there is no more or less water in the blood than is ideal, and no more or less of each given hormone. Blood sugar is no exception; in order to avoid potentially dangerous extremes, the body rapidly compensates for any changes in blood sugar levels caused by food intake (or stress, as we shall explore in Chapter 2) or a skipped meal.

Ideally, blood sugar levels should fall slightly a few hours after a meal (thus triggering hunger) and rise as the digested meal passes into the bloodstream. However, many people's blood sugar levels rise and fall dramatically throughout the day. When blood sugar plummets, mood swings, irritability, anxiety, lethargy, sleepiness and cravings can set in, and perhaps even palpitations, headaches or light-headedness. These symptoms of low blood sugar prompt you to react in quick-fix survival mode; it is imperative that the body gets its blood sugar levels up fast or it could slump into a hypoglycaemic (low blood sugar) coma, so any good intentions can go straight out of the window as you reach for that habitual biscuit, cake, chocolate bar, sugary drink or even a stimulant like caffeine or a cigarette (discussed in Chapter 2) to provide the rapid fix you need.

Meanwhile, your body is busy taking its own urgent steps in order to get blood sugar levels back within the ideal parameters. It rapidly releases stores of glucose and, at the same time, pumps out adrenaline to make sure the fuel gets around the body as quickly as possible, which means that low blood sugar is a direct stress on the body.

THE BLOOD SUGAR ROLLERCOASTER RIDE

The dotted wavy line in the diagram opposite represents normal, healthy fluctuations in blood sugar levels that occur over a period of a few hours or a whole day, depending on your metabolism and diet. The straight zigzag line represents undesirable extreme rises and falls in blood sugar levels caused by a diet that throws the body's natural equilibrium out of kilter. If you notice that you are suddenly feeling tired and low, struggling to concentrate and craving sweet, starchy food, you are probably experiencing a blood sugar drop. A common reaction is to grab a sugary snack, which, combined with your body's own efforts to resolve the crisis (see page 14), causes blood sugar levels to rise sharply. You may briefly feel better, but this sudden rise is quickly followed by another dramatic fall and then the whole cycle begins again. This may occur twice during the day – mid-morning and mid-evening are often marked by drops in blood sugar levels, especially if your breakfast and lunch are composed mainly of fast-releasing foods (see box, page 21) – or it may occur as often as once an hour, if you regularly snack on fast-releasing foods.

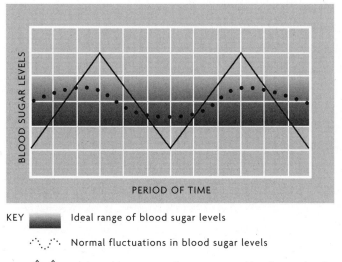

KEY   Ideal range of blood sugar levels

Normal fluctuations in blood sugar levels

Undesirable extreme fluctuations in blood sugar levels

The sugar cravings cycle

If sugar is so harmful, why do we love it so much and even crave it? On the most basic level, our brains demand a constant supply of fuel and if they don't receive it, we can crave sugar as a quick-fix survival response – to help us 'normalize'. When we eat sugar, therefore, we are fulfilling the brain's need to receive a non-stop supply of glucose and we feel good, even settled, where we might have felt agitation before.

However, the relief from the slump lasts only for a short while because rather than raising blood sugar levels to within the desirable parameters, our 'quick fix' often pushes them beyond the ideal maximum. This is caused by a combination of the means we use – the chocolate, coffee, cigarette – and a by-now confused and over-reacting body. In order to deal with the sudden excess in blood sugar, the body overcompensates with the release of too much insulin in one burst that then sends blood sugar levels crashing, leaving you craving yet another fix. It is a confusing, exhausting and mood-upsetting vicious cycle.

Our relationship and intake of sweet foods is complex and often conditioned from childhood, as we will expolre further in later chapters.

How do we balance our energy for the brain?

The brain can demand around 20 per cent of the body's total energy output when in a resting state, but this can rise to 70–80 per cent when we are in a stressed, protective mode. Ideally we receive this as glucose from the slow release of carbohydrates from any plant food we eat: vegetables, fruit, nuts, seeds, grains or beans – or lactose in dairy. All of these provide a more stable delivery of glucose to the bloodstream and therefore the brain. The word carbohydrate has recently been used more casually in the context of low-carb diets, and the media refer to starchy carbohydrates, those mostly in grains, beans and root vegetables, but they are found throughout all plant foods that we eat. Starchy carbs can also provoke a high insulin response when they feature too highly in our diets so they can also contribute to blood sugar imbalance.

These natural food sources are complex carbohydrates, so they take time to break down with digestion. More 'simple' carbohydrates break down into their component sugars quicker and, hence, taste sweeter. Simple carbohydrates are those found in pure sugar, fruit sugar (fructose) and other sweeteners, but also in refined or 'white' products such as white flours, white rice and white pasta – so not wholegrain where the outer, fibrous hull of the grain is retained and slows down sugar release into the bloodstream.

What foods should I cut back on or avoid?

So how can you ensure that your body receives the sugar it needs without sending your blood sugar levels into an exhausting and damaging soar-and-slump pattern? An awareness of which foods perpetuate blood sugar highs and lows will allow you to be more in control of how you feel. As these extreme trajectories take with them your moods and energy, it is best to reduce these foods overall in your diet and avoid making snacking on sweets a habit.

This can be a little uncomfortable as we change our tastes and our brain shifts (see Chapter 2), but a sweet tooth can be reconditioned so that we can then enjoy these sugary foods as an occasional treat that won't rule our choices and behaviours. When we make changes, it is important to pay mindful attention to the quality of our energy and mood that we feel as a result. Noticing the changes in our body helps us become more in tune with what makes us feel jangly and excited, rather than the more sustained nourishment that leaves us with more mental clarity and a sense of satisfaction.

Of course, while it is easy to spot sugar in a biscuit, a bar of chocolate, a packet of sweets, a milkshake or a doughnut, there are other foods in which it is hard to detect. More insidious are the hidden quantities of sugar contained in less obviously sweetened foods: bread, baked beans and other canned foods, fruit yoghurt, fruit juices, breakfast cereals, ketchup and other sauces or dressings, as well as many ready-made meals. Once you become aware of this, you can see how the amount of sugar you are eating each day can easily creep up without you even realizing it. That is why it is a good idea to eat as many fresh, unprocessed foods as possible and to eat artificially sweetened foods only in small amounts.

Check the backs of a few packets in supermarkets and see how high sugar comes in the list of ingredients. Manufacturers have many ways of fooling us about the sugar content of foods, hiding it in fruit 'flavoured' products, even those marketed as health foods:

Barley malt	Fruit juice concentrate	Maple syrup
Beet sugar	Invert sugar	Microcrystalline cellulose
Brown rice syrup	Lactose (from milk)	Molasses
Brown sugar	Galatose (from milk)	Polydextrose
Cane juice	Glucose	Raisin juice
Corn sweetener	Granulated sugar	Raisin syrup
Corn syrup	High-fructose corn syrup	Raw sugar
Date sugar	Honey	Sucrose
Demarera sugar	Malted barley	Unrefined sugar
Dextrin	Maltodextrin	White sugar
Dextrose	Maltose	Agave syrup
Fructose (from fruits)	Mannitol, sorbitol, xylitol	

Fresh fruit, the healthier sweet option?

If a label says in the nutritional analysis that the food contains more than 10g of 'carbohydrates, of which sugars', this means it has sugar in excess of what we need. However, although fruit will always contain more sugar than this, it comes in a naturally complex form with a whole host of nutrients that help our body to process the sugar with minimum damage. We crave the sweetness of fruit because it leads us to the high vitamin C content, but we have learned to keep the sweetness and throw away the protective package.

If your blood sugar levels are poorly balanced, even foods that are from natural sources, such as fruit juices or dried fruits, can create havoc in your body. These foods are close to the form they came in from nature but have been processed by humans so the sugar is more concentrated – a glass of orange juice can have as much sugar as the equivalent amount in a soda drink. It is therefore best to dilute any juices with 70 per cent water and to eat dried fruits accompanied by some protein (to slow their sugar release into the bloodstream), such as a handful of nuts or yoghurt. Fresh fruit is always a good dietary option, though, and is best to turn to for a 'healthy' sweet treat rather than dried fruit or juices.

What is your diet doing to your blood sugar levels?

One of the main reasons why specific foods, certain eating patterns or missing meals affect the way you feel is that they have an impact on your blood sugar levels. So what actually happens?

Eating slow-releasing carbohydrates:	Glucose from carbohydrates takes time to be broken down and reach the bloodstream, so blood sugar rises gradually over a few hours.
Eating proteins or fats with carbohydrates:	Slows down the breakdown of carbohydrates in a meal, so blood sugar rises slowly over a few hours.
Eating sugary foods/fast-releasing carbohydrates/sugary drinks:	Blood sugar rises within minutes, followed by a dramatic fall.
Drinking caffeine:	Blood sugar rises rapidly, creating a stimulant effect followed by a slump (see page 50–1).
Drinking alcohol, particularly on an empty stomach:	Blood sugar rises initially and falls rapidly.
Missing a meal:	Blood sugar drops. Missing breakfast can have a dramatic effect because of the long gap between dinner today and lunch tomorrow.

The Glycaemic Index

By choosing your food carefully, you can largely avoid steep rises in blood sugar. The glycaemic index (GI) has been devised as a method of defining food according to the speed at which it is digested and released into the bloodstream as glucose. The more fibre, protein and fat that is eaten alongside starchy or sugary foods, the more slowly those foods are digested and released as sugar into your system. Rice cakes, for example, are very fast-releasing – they have a high GI score. However, when spread with houmous, which is rich in protein and fat, the GI is reduced. The table here gives the GI of various common foods.

GLYCAEMIC INDEX OF FOODS

Slow-releasing foods	Moderate-releasing	Fast-releasing
• fish/seafood • meat/poultry • eggs • whole milk/whole milk yoghurt • cheese • soy/tofu • seeds/nuts • tahini/houmous • green vegetables • peas/beans/pulses • tomatoes • mushrooms • raw root vegetables, such as carrots/beetroot • boiled sweet potato • grapefruit • plums • apples • pears • oranges • whole grains	• whole rye bread/rye crackers • muesli • barley • basmati rice • buckwheat • pitta bread/wholemeal bread • pineapple • melon • honey • cooked root vegetables – carrots • new potatoes • raisins • skimmed milk/low-fat yoghurt	• baked beans • white rice • white bread • parsnips • processed cereals, especially cornflakes • mashed/baked potato/French fries • baked sweet potato • cooked root vegetables – beetroot, parsnip, turnip • watermelon • cornflakes • rice cakes • white bread • white and brown rice • sweetcorn • bananas • dried fruit • apricots • mangoes • honey

For a more even release of glucose into the bloodstream, minimize your intake of high GI (fast-releasing) foods, and eat them in combination with low GI (slow-releasing) foods, for example:

- Brown rice with stir-fried chicken and green vegetables.
- A baked potato with tuna and salad.
- A banana with a handful of pumpkin seeds.

- Rye or sourdough toast with poached eggs.
- Muesli with yoghurt.
- Rice cakes with tahini or houmous.

Fibre plays a vital role in the management of blood sugar, hence the foundation for blood sugar balance is plenty of vegetables and naturally sweet foods such as fruit. The higher the a food's fibre content, the lower its GI score is likely to be.

Do I need supplements to support my diet?

In addition to eating low GI foods or slow-releasing combinations, certain nutrients are necessary for the processes that regulate blood sugar levels. We can obtain many of these from a varied diet (see food sources on pages 84–6), but stress, modern distribution methods and processing of foods can mean we take on less than we need to function optimally, even if we are getting the minimum recommended amount. The following are found in a good multivitamin and mineral supplement (ask in a healthfood shop) or dedicated glucose regulation formulas:

- The mineral chromium is of key importance, as it appears to be involved in the insulin mechanism. Many people find it helpful to take 100mcg of chromium at breakfast (often within a multivitamin and mineral supplement) and lunch while they are supporting blood sugar changes, because it may help reduce cravings.
- Another mineral, magnesium, is essential for the conversion of glucose to the form it is stored as, and vice versa. Ideal forms of magnesium to use are magnesium citrate or magnesium ascorbate, a type of vitamin C that helps support the adrenal glands. These are likely to be working overtime if your blood sugar levels are all over the place, as we discuss in the next chapter. Magnesium pantothenate is

a combination of the mineral and vitamin B5, another good adrenal nutrient. (More on magnesium on pages 54–5.)

- The B vitamins, particularly B3, but also B1 and B2, are needed for the processing of sugar in the body and all are best taken as part of a multivitamin or B-complex tablet.
- Vanadium and manganese are minerals that are involved in the way the body deals with glucose. They are needed in only very small amounts, so are best included in a multivitamin blend rather than taken separately.
- Other factors that support blood sugar balance and may be found in supplements are: cinnamon (see page 28), alpha-lipoic acid, green tea extract and fenugreek.

These nutrients are found within a diet that includes masses of green leafy vegetables, fruit, nuts, seeds, fish, eggs and whole grains, but stress uses them up at a great rate. A nutritionist will be able to help you work out which supplements would be best for your individual needs.

Are you really hungry?

Your blood sugar levels will be more stable if you eat regularly, but although the advice is given to eat 'little and often', this can be a double-edged sword. Yes, continually putting food into our mouths will ensure our blood sugar never gets the chance to drop, but it also sets us up to become fixated on eating constantly, confuses our relationship with hunger and when we truly need food, and is a strain on the digestive system, which needs periods where each section of the digestive tract can rest and heal. Constantly having to digest food as we start the process from the beginning again also demands an awful lot of energy.

Eating when we feel properly hungry is the best way for our bodies to receive food. If we've had years of blood sugar imbalance (and most modern days are set up this way), regular mealtimes help create a framework from which to begin. Rather than constantly snacking, you can then see if you need a well-timed, well-chosen snack to support blood sugar levels. For instance, you may struggle going more than four hours without food, so you will need a mid-afternoon snack to tide you over for the journey home from work and give you the resources to be able to choose and prepare an evening meal that fulfills your needs – something with protein and vegetables rather than a knee-jerk big bowl of starchy carbs like pasta because you've hit a blood sugar low.

We'll go through some specifics within the recipes, so you can explore what suits you best.

Good mood mornings

The word breakfast comes from breaking your overnight fast – providing the body with fuel first thing in the morning to get it going for the day. Skipping the most important meal of the day sets the scene for fluctuating blood sugar levels, because by lunchtime the brain hasn't had a direct fuel delivery since dinner the night before. So always have breakfast, even if it's not as soon as you get up. You can build up to a proper meal if this is a new habit, 'weaning' your body onto food so it gets used to receiving it at this time. If you felt the symptoms listed at the beginning of this section were very familiar, you may find this little change to your routine makes a big difference.

Very Berry Smoothie

Although this delightful smoothie is best made in the summer, using fresh berries, it's also good in the winter with frozen ones. Fruits such as apples, berries or plums are the better choice over less tart fruits if you are craving sweetness, and if this doesn't seem sweet enough for you at first, you'll notice that tastes change quickly. Berries in particular have been shown to reduce sugar spikes after meals, so they are also a great alternative to wean you off sweet puddings.

The yoghurt, avocado and flaxseed oil provide protein and healthy fats to help blood sugar balance and create satisfaction at the beginning of the day. Feel free to vary the ingredients as suits.

Serves 2

6 tablespoons mixed berries, such as blueberries, strawberries, raspberries, blackcurrants, blackberries

6 tablespoons live, plain yoghurt or coconut yoghurt

½ avocado

2 dessertspoons organic flaxseed oil

I   Put all the ingredients in a blender for 1 minute and whizz until combined. Pour into a glass and drink immediately.

Scrambled Eggs on Rye with Leeks and Mushrooms

Eggs are the most bioavailable protein we can eat and as such they help to balance blood sugar and also support brain chemistry, as we will discuss later on in this book. This is a densely satisfying breakfast that will help reset appetite and energy for the coming day; it's well worth cooking, even if you can only manage to make this at weekends. You could substitute eggs for smoked salmon if you prefer, and if you are vegan, a nut burger or tofu scramble can provide the protein part.

Rye bread has been shown to be particularly good for balancing blood sugar and slow-release energy. As an alternative to wheat, it still has a little of the gluten that may contribute to digestive upset and mood issues (see the digestive connection to mental health in Chapter 5) but if you use a sourdough bread, this process aids in the breaking down this sticky protein and even helps the health of our gut environment. This is true in wheat bread, too.

A savoury breakfast can be helpful to those with sweet cravings, as it does not set off these urges first thing, delaying the inevitable reaching for a biscuit . . . Leek and mushrooms are used here, but you could substitute them with spinach, avocado, watercress, cucumber, tomatoes or any vegetable that provides extra minerals and fibre.

Serves 2

4 eggs

dash of milk or almond milk

I teaspoon olive oil

I large leek, sliced

8 chestnut mushrooms, sliced

I tablespoon chopped parsley
   (optional)

2 slices rye sourdough bread

I teaspoon butter, plus a little
   extra for buttering

pinch of salt (ideally a sea salt
   and herbs blend) and freshly
   ground black pepper

1   Beat the eggs in a bowl with a dash of milk or almond milk, freshly ground black pepper and a pinch of salt.

2   Heat the olive oil in a large saucepan and, on a low heat, start to gently cook the leek and mushrooms.

3   Some people don't like parsley with their eggs, but if this combination appeals to you, add freshly chopped parsley to the leeks and mushrooms just before you've finished cooking them to give the meal a green freshness.

4   When the leeks and mushrooms are almost done, put the bread in the toaster and quickly heat the butter in a separate pan. Add the eggs and stir constantly on a very low heat until they are the texture you like.

5   When the leeks and mushrooms are softened but not browned serve them on two plates. Butter the toast lightly, put it on the plates next to the leeks and mushrooms and top with the eggs.

Apple Porridge

Porridge has a reputation for being the perfect breakfast food. Oats do not contain any gluten and have a slightly higher fat content than other grains, so they release their sugars much slower and they take longer to digest. They don't contain much protein, so adding nuts and seeds – and almond milk – helps their blood sugar balancing potential.

Here much of the sweetness comes from cinnamon, a truly helpful start to the day for blood sugar maintenance; this spice contains a bioflavonoid called MHCP that mimics insulin, actively moving sugar into cells for energy. A teaspoon a day has been shown to help balance blood sugar levels, even in people with diabetes. It is highly effective at telling the brain that you have eaten something sweet with positive rather than negative consequences, but you may want to start with the honey included here, then slowly bring down the amount as your taste buds adapt to reduced sweetness. Cinnamon can also be added to coffee, tea, yoghurt, berries and curries, and it is also found in many herbal tea blends.

Serves 2

5 heaped tablespoons rolled oats
almond milk, to taste
1 apple, grated
½ teaspoon honey (optional –
 can be reduced or
 replaced with coconut, see
 page 39)

½ teaspoon ground cinnamon
1 dessertspoon ground High-
 Five Seeds (page 57) or any
 mix of raw nuts

1   Put the oats into a pan, cover with cold water and cook over a
    low heat, stirring gently. As the oats begin to absorb the water,
    slowly add small amounts of milk, stirring all the time, until the
    porridge is the consistency you like. When the oats are cooked –
    this should take about 5 minutes – stir in the grated apple, honey
    (if using) and cinnamon, sprinkle the seed blend or nuts over the
    top and serve immediately.

Getting into the food rhythm of the day...

After a satisfying breakfast, hopefully you will feel more able to sustain your energy levels and good mood until lunchtime. This shift away from the often-usual modern pattern of eating the biggest proportion of food towards the end of the day (when we're more likely to store it overnight as fat) can prevent us running on stress hormones for fuel (see next chapter) and instead on food that has been broken down and slowly released. Lunch and dinner can be made from similar ingredients, but whenever possible, having lunch as the larger feast helps us to fall in line with our metabolic design. When we sustain ourselves from the morning, it can start to feel more natural to have a lighter evening meal and fewer cravings (see Chapter 9 for examples of daily meal plans to help).

Salad Dressings

With a great dressing even the humblest of salad vegetables can be taken out of the fridge and quickly turned into a feast, which means you will be more motivated and find it easier and tastier to simply include oceans of leaves and other veg in your diet. The best way to make these dressings is to put all the ingredients into a jar and shake well. The dressings will keep in the fridge in a sealed jar for about a week.

These dressings contain ingredients with significant health potential; lemon helps the digestion of food, garlic supports circulation and immunity, while olive oil is anti-inflammatory. Every one of these dressings provides a host of antioxidants that protect tissues from damage.

Creamy Vinaigrette

6 tablespoons olive oil
2 tablespoons balsamic vinegar
1 heaped teaspoon wholegrain
    mustard
freshly ground black pepper

Tangy Vinaigrette

6 tablespoons olive oil
2 tablespoons lemon juice
1 heaped teaspoon smooth
    green-peppercorn mustard
1 clove garlic, crushed
pinch of salt

Oriental Bite

3 tablespoons olive oil
1 dessertspoon sesame oil
juice of 2 limes
1 dessertspoon chopped
    coriander/cilantro
3 dashes of Tabasco sauce

Rich Pesto Dressing

1 teaspoon pesto
4 tablespoons olive oil
juice of ½ lemon
pinch of salt and freshly ground
    black pepper

Proper Green Salad

Creating lunch and dinner around plants as often as possible provides the equivalent of the green leaves that would probably have made up most of our ancestors' diets. This is the healthiest way that we can receive our mainstay carbohydrate sources, especially from cruciferous vegetables (broccoli, cabbage, pak choi, cauliflower, kale, mustard greens) to supply trace minerals, soluble fibre and slow-release energy for blood sugar balance.

A salad like this is the basis of a meal, to which a protein part – fish, eggs, meat, beans, tofu, nuts, goat's cheese, etc. – can be added. If you're having a side of a starchy carbohydrate for energy, this is best added at lunchtime (especially for weight maintenance) so you use up that dense energy as fuel in the afternoon. Best-choice starches are brown basmati rice, sweet potatoes, buckwheat pasta or noodles and quinoa.

Salad dressings provide an oil base that allows us to absorb the fat-soluble nutrients such as vitamins A and E, and the immune-supportive antioxidant carotenoids that give leaves and other veg their bright colours.

Serves 4

2 generous handfuls of baby
  spinach
4 broccoli florets, trimmed
2 tablespoons white cabbage,
  shredded
1 handful of watercress

1 handful of sprouted alfalfa
1 handful of sprouted mung
  beans
5 cm (2 inches) cucumber, diced
1 tablespoon pumpkin seeds

1 Toss all the ingredients together in a large bowl and serve with
   one of the salad dressings on page 31. If you think there may be
   any leftovers, dress the salad on individual plates rather than in
   the large serving bowl to prevent it going soggy.

Baby Spinach and Goat's Cheese Salad

Here is an example of a really quick salad you can throw together, especially when you have one of your home-made, ready-prepared dressings (see page 31). It includes leaves, protein from the goat's cheese and nuts and with the High-Five Seeds topping (see page 57) or walnuts, you're getting a good dose of essential fatty acids, too.

Serves 2

250 g (9 oz) baby spinach leaves, washed

150 g (5 oz) goat's cheese, such as feta, crumbled

3 tablespoons Creamy or Tangy Vinaigrette (see page 31)

2 dessertspoons ground High-Five Seeds (see page 57) or nuts, e.g. walnuts

1 In a large salad bowl, toss the spinach with the crumbled goat's cheese and vinaigrette and sprinkle with the seeds or nuts.

Quinoa with Roasted Vegetables

Quinoa is unusually high in protein for a grain, and it can also be categorized as a seed, with the healthy oil content that it brings; all highly supportive for blood sugar balance and consistent brain energy. It was revered by the Aztecs as the 'mother grain'. For vegans it is an important ingredient that can be loaded up with vegetables to make a complete meal. It also works well as an alternative to pasta for those who do not tolerate wheat, and is great for a packed lunch.

Serves 4

1 red pepper, and sliced
1 green pepper, and sliced
2 red onions, sliced
2 courgettes/zucchini, sliced
2 Portobello mushrooms, sliced
8–10 cherry tomatoes
8–10 cloves garlic

olive oil, for drizzling
a few sprigs of fresh thyme
170 g/6 oz/1 cup quinoa
480 ml/16 fl oz/2 mugs of water
sea salt and freshly ground black pepper

1   Preheat the oven to 180°C/350°F/Gas Mark 4.
2   Toss all the vegetables together in a large roasting tin/pan with plenty of olive oil and the thyme. Season with salt and pepper.
3   Roast in the oven for 30–40 minutes, or until all the vegetables are soft and turning brown at the edges.
4   Meanwhile, rinse the quinoa thoroughly and put it in a saucepan with the water. (If quinoa is not rinsed well, it can be a bit bitter.) Bring to the boil, then cover and turn down to a simmer until it is cooked – this should take about 15 minutes. Serve a mound of quinoa topped with a selection of the vegetables and drizzled with a little olive oil.

Crunchy Oaty Crumble

Sometimes we need a treat or it is an occasion that deserves a dessert. When we don't have sweet treats all the time, we can appreciate and enjoy them without expecting one after every meal. The desserts in this book all have properties that help support, rather than work against, the factors that balance blood sugar, particularly after a meal rich in protein. This pudding is particularly helpful as you'll see it contains all of the elements we've discussed as being supportive for energy and mood. This is important to be able to enjoy it without the guilt or self-criticism that can upset blood sugar balance through internally-generated stress.

You can replace the apples with any of your favourite fruits, or add blackberries or blackcurrants for extra proanthocyanadins, the purple-coloured chemicals that also help regulate blood sugar.

Serves 4

500 g (1 lb 2 oz) muesli or
   rolled oats

2 teaspoons ground cinnamon

2 tablespoons pumpkin seeds

about 10 walnuts, roughly
   chopped

40 g (1½ oz) cold butter, cut into
   cubes

3 large cooking apples, peeled,
   cored and sliced

2 tablespoons raisins or sultanas/
   golden raisins

1 tablespoon brown sugar

vanilla yoghurt (see page 38),
   Greek or coconut yoghurt
   (see page 39), to serve

1   Preheat the oven to 180°C/350°F/Gas Mark 4.

2   Put the muesli or oats plus 1 teaspoon of the cinnamon,
    the pumpkin seeds and the broken-up walnuts into a large
    mixing bowl with the butter. Mix with your fingers until there
    are no lumps of butter left. Alternatively, you can melt the
    butter and mix it in that way. Lay the apples in a baking dish,
    sprinkled with the raisins, remaining cinnamon and sugar.
    Add 4 tablespoons of water.

3   Evenly scatter the crumble mixture over the top of the apples
    so that they are well covered. Bake in the oven for about
    40 minutes, or until the apples are soft when skewered.

4   Serve with vanilla yoghurt (see page 38), Greek or coconut
    yoghurt (see page 39).

Craving-busting snacks to avoid blood sugar lows

We typically have a blood sugar low at 4pm, when traditionally the tea and cakes are wheeled out. A snack at this time or just before can help you to resist this instant gratification and allow you to feel you are not at the mercy of cravings caused by blood sugar rollercoasters.

Fresh nuts and seeds

Nuts and seeds are perfect little nutritional packages, containing protein, starchy carbohydrates, essential oils and micro-nutrients such as B vitamins, magnesium and zinc – everything a plant needs to grow. It is good to have them on hand for when sugar cravings strike. Best choices are fresh almonds, hazelnuts, cashews or Brazils – avoid nuts that are roasted or salted. For seeds, have a mixture of pumpkin, sunflower and sesame; mix them up as you like and carry them in a small container, perhaps with a small proportion of dried fruit to help sate a sweet craving. Chew them well to digest them fully and acknowledge your body receiving them so you feel satisfied and are not tempted to eat more than you need to.

Fresh fruit with plain yoghurt

Accompanied by a small pot or a couple of tablespoons of plain yoghurt, fruit makes a satisfying mini-meal. Choose berries and cherries in the summer, juicy ripe pears and a variety of apples in the winter, or any fruit you fancy for this dish. Bananas and grapes are a good choice for those with blood sugar issues as they are particularly sweet, so they are an ideal treat to sate a craving, but only eat them occasionally because they have a high sugar content.

Greek yoghurt is the best choice of all yoghurts, having a higher protein and lower lactose (milk sugar) level – choose plain and organic, and full-fat helps balance blood sugar and satisfy appetite more than processed, low-fat kinds. If you don't tolerate dairy, choose coconut yoghurt rather than soy, which is highly processed and may disrupt hormones.

If you want to satisfy a sweet tooth, rather than adding sugars like honey or agave, try adding berries, unsweetened coconut, ground almonds, natural vanilla essence and unsweetened apple purée. Coconut provides a natural sweetness and contains plant saturated fats called medium-chain triglycerides (MCTs) that help satisfy any need for sugar as they provide a dense energy source. Use as unsweetened desiccated coconut or flakes.

You could include a few pieces of dried fruit, but remember they are a very concentrated form of sugar and should be eaten in only small amounts. Buy unsulphured varieties from healthfood shops as the sulphur preservatives can irritate the digestive system and cause bloating.

Which lifestyle changes best balance blood sugar?

In the next chapter we will examine the effects of stress on mood and mental health. As much of this relationship is wrapped up in blood sugar regulation, lifestyle measures to allow mind-body relaxation and to help us cope with life's demands are most crucial for blood sugar balance. We will also explore further ideas and advice in Chapter 6 on Appetite Regulation.

TOP TIPS TO REGULATE
BLOOD SUGAR BALANCE

- Always eat breakfast, building it up as you get used to the new habit – even some fruit or a handful of nuts can help.
- Eat regular meals, noting when you actually feel hungry and when you feel full.
- Include well-timed snacks, if needed.
- Include fibre- and protein-rich foods in each meal.
- Avoid sugar, foods containing sugar, and honey; save dried and fresh fruits as occasional treats or cut them out entirely if that helps you stay away. Note: you may feel low in energy and experience feelings of 'detox', such as irritability or headaches, as you reduce sugar levels – see Chapter 6 on Appetite Regulation for more information.
- Look at labels on food products for hidden sugars in the ingredients and a 'carbohydrates of which sugars' content of over 10 g/¼ oz per 100 g/3½ oz.
- Reduce or avoid refined foods (white bread, white rice, etc.), processed and fast foods.
- Dilute fruit or vegetable juices with 70 per cent water, or just have water.
- Eat dried fruit with protein, such as plain yoghurt or a handful of nuts.
- Consider taking nutritional supplements designed to support blood sugar balance.

Part Two

RECIPES FOR SELF-SOOTHING

CHAPTER 2

CALMING AN
ANXIOUS MIND

We all know that a stressful event affects immediate mood, so it is no surprise that ongoing or chronic stress can have far-reaching consequences for our mental health. We can find ourselves less tolerant, less adaptable and more easily agitated when life's challenges build up. The stress response is an immediate survival strategy, and for us humans the brain is the main organ of survival.

We have a large reliance on thinking our way out of danger, but we also experience the heightened sensory acuity that comes with being on high alert. Not only do we see and hear more sensitively to be aware of threat, but our minds go into hyper-vigilant mode. This can have us scanning our environment constantly, running through possible scenarios in our heads, worrying about negative outcomes and even unable to see any bright side; this 'catastrophizing' is a survival strategy we can learn from a young age to keep us 'safe' in the only way we know how. It can become a habit as we get older and get stuck in a mental rut. If we grew up feeling unsafe, this way in which we view the world can prompt us to live in this 'constant alert' of the stress response and find it difficult to come down from this state, maybe experiencing this as agitation, panic, anxiety, fear or a sense of being overwhelmed.

As mentioned in relation to blood sugar, in this state our brain demands up to three times more energy than when we are calm. Nutritional support is key for providing these nutrients needed for energy, but also to help us cope with stress and therefore sparing this high need. This can also help soothe the cravings and food impulses that can accompany stress and create a vicious cycle of dietary habits that do not support our ability to cope in these situations. Some specific nutritional considerations and foods can also actively soothe an agitated nervous system.

Stress that persists (even low level when continual) results in low moods, fatigue and increased susceptibility to illness. It is important for us to be able to recognize when we are near to or have crossed the point at which it is overwhelming to be able to look after ourselves.

On the list below, tick the symptoms that apply to you regularly:

- Easily angered or irritable.
- Feeling as though you can't cope.
- Exhaustion.
- Difficulty making decisions.
- Lacking motivation.
- Mood swings.
- Over-reacting to life's everyday stresses.
- Difficulty sleeping.
- Waking up anxious.
- Panic attacks.
- Feeling particularly groggy when you wake up in the morning.

If you ticked six or more of the above symptoms, your body may be struggling to deal with stress.

Why do I feel this way?

It is important to state that stress is not simply a 'bad thing', rather it describes anything that creates a heightened response in us. We need this to a degree to keep us motivated and interested, and it naturally occurs when we have the focus and new brain pathways of learning a new task, skill or system. This is called 'eustress' and describes a challenge that can strengthen and sharpen systems, such as brain-teasing puzzles or weight-bearing exercise where bone growth is provoked by the stress of force upon it.

However, stress becomes detrimental when it is relentless, ongoing and has an underlying and pervading sense of being 'unsafe', when we feel we have no control in the outcome or cannot see an endpoint. We play out the survival fight-flight-freeze responses with a full mind-body response. Even if we are simply worrying, are in emotional turmoil or anxious about a deadline, our heart pumps faster, our pupils dilate and our minds race or freeze. As survival is only concerned with short-term immediate safety, blood and oxygen is rerouted away from digestion, skin and reproductive organs – more long-term concerns. They are then delivered to the brain for quick decision-making, and to muscle, ready for action or immobilisation (the latter common in those with trauma). If we go towards fight, this may play out in the modern world as irritation, anger or intolerance. Flight can become withdrawal, storming out or avoidance.

The fight-or-flight part is fuelled by adrenaline produced by the adrenal glands. Freeze states are older, more primitive brain responses that also involve the gut (more in Chapter 4). These days, unlike for our hunter-gatherer ancestors, we rarely escape stress by fighting or fleeing. We often face ongoing stress factors that cause our bodies to release adrenaline almost constantly, leading to a vicious cycle of permanently taut muscles, pent-up tension and a racing, constantly vigilant mind.

Another stress hormone released by the adrenals is cortisol. Under normal circumstances, cortisol is released on a daily cycle whereby it is higher in the morning, making us feel more alert, and lower at night, helping us to sleep. However, when you have been stressed for some time, this rhythm is disrupted; cortisol stays high to take over from the initial rush of adrenaline if our mind-bodies perceive there is ongoing 'danger', even if this is relationship issues or an excessive to-do list. This in turn affects sleep patterns and energy levels and ultimately can make you demotivated. When this downward spiral pushes you over the line of where you feel you can cope, 'stress related' symptoms often occur, such as anxiety, IBS, insomnia, lower back and shoulder pain, headaches, teeth grinding, skin issues and more.

The stress of stimulants

It is also important that you limit your intake of 'stimulants' – such as sugar and sugary foods or drinks, refined foods (including biscuits or white bread), coffee, tea, alcohol and cigarettes – which trigger the body's stress response by provoking a sudden, dramatic rise in blood sugar levels. Stimulants include alcohol, caffeine, nicotine and recreational drugs. If you have an addictive relationships to any of these, rather than going straight into full avoidance of them, begin to address sugar and your stress issues first by reducing them gradually, at a rate that makes you feel comfortable.

What's the link with my diet?

One of the first body mechanisms to fall prey to prolonged stress is blood sugar balance, as the body systems involved in blood sugar regulation can easily become exhausted. This is a chicken-and-egg situation:

- When falling blood sugar levels are making constant demands on them, the adrenal glands (there is one of these on top of each kidney) soon become burnt out (see below) and are no longer able to perform their job efficiently. They adapt by rewiring the body into a 'hyper' state, where even if the original external stressor disappears, your body may well remain in alarm mode.
- When blood sugar levels drop, there are only a few ways to bring them back up again to where we can feel 'normal' and function – food, stimulants or stress hormones from the adrenal glands. Because the fight-or-flight response needs immediate energy, sugar is released from glycogen stores in the liver and muscle. We can become accustomed to running on adrenaline and we lose hunger signals, for example, if we frequently skip breakfast and rush out of the door in a high-stress state, it can then feel 'normal' to energize ourselves via stress, but that will eventually wear us out and keep our brains highly agitated.

The nutritional advice given here builds on that from the previous chapter; blood sugar balance is foundational for allowing us to cope with stress and place minimum strain on the adrenal glands. When blood sugar levels are low, brain chemicals responsible for motivation and focus, such as serotonin and dopamine, fall, so until this mechanism is brought back into an even rhythm, it is difficult to break the stress cycle (this is discussed in more detail in the next chapter). It can take time and dedicated self-care to regenerate tired adrenals and find equilibrium, but as well as the protein-rich foods we need to slow down the rate at which sugar is released into the bloodstream, and need in some specific help for adrenal support and self-soothing body processes.

Sugar and stress – a hidden secret

Sugar craving is part and parcel of the stress response, especially when chronic stress or trauma has led to fatigue, when we turn to the hit of sweet foods simply to keep going, but then we get caught in the cycle of highs and lows described in Chapter 1. Regardless of how we might be trying to avoid eating sugary foods for our health, when we go into that survival response, immediate need trumps any long-term healthy plans. When stress, worry or overload hit, we move into impulsive mode and we respond to signals to 'fuel-up!' Another vicious cycle can be formed here, as we then feel angry at ourselves for having no willpower, which in turn adds the stress of feeling guilt or shame.

It is helpful to understand how it is an automatic response that we can crave sugar when stressed and from there try not to beat ourselves up, but rather use this information to notice when things have become too much and support ourselves through nutrition and lifestyle. When we consider that our first food, breast milk, was sweet (from the only sugar in the animal – not plant – kingdom that we eat, lactose) and this would be associated with the warmth and safety of a mother or other caregiver, we can see we are set up to self-soothe through sugar from the offset. As babies we were dependent on another to provide this nourishment, which came with a rush of the 'love hormone' oxytocin, which creates a strong sense of wellbeing. We can use sugar to try to recreate this feeling when our brains feel agitated or overwhelmed. When we add in that as children many of us were given sweets or desserts as comfort – 'have this biscuit to make you feel better' – or reward – 'if you eat your vegetables, you can have some ice cream' – we can see that the stage is set to turn straight to cakes, chocolate or cookies to settle and soothe.

All of this is a response to the hit that eating sugar brings. There is much debate around the question of whether sugar is an addictive substance, but those who have been in its throes will agree that it is extremely hard to give up, especially in times of worry, fear, challenge or overwork. Eating sugar provokes a rush of the neurotransmitter dopamine, which is released to give us a happy feeling as a reward when we do anything that promotes survival of the species – eating, exercise, having sex – but also we are group animals, laughter, hugs, dancing, singing and being with those we feel safe with. When we don't have enough of these in life, we can seek out alternate dopamine sources, such as sugar, but also excessive or addictive tendencies that produce this same 'lift' in mood. Of course, this comes with the high, followed by the low, reminding us that finding the middle ground in blood sugar and lifestyle choices can also help stabilize mood.

Of all the substances in the human diet, sugar is the most insidious. It is estimated that our hunter-gatherer ancestors ate 20 teaspoons of sugar a year from natural carbohydrate sources, while modern man consumes nearly twice that daily, from refined sources such as cakes, biscuits, sweets, sodas and fruit juices. Sugar consumption is the number one dietary concern associated with mental health issues and depletes nutrients such as B vitamins and magnesium needed for optimal brain function; it is estimated that 1 molecule of sugar eaten uses up 56 molecules of magnesium in its metabolism (see more on magnesium and stress below).

Bringing down sugar consumption can take time after years of irregularities and needs to be done with care – especially during times of stress – allowing a period of adjustment where cravings may heighten as brain chemistry readjusts. The work on sugar addiction by the late researcher Bart Hoebel showed that rats given the choice between sugar and cocaine overwhelmingly chose the sugar, even when the cocaine dose offered was raised.

With sugar provoking a dopamine response, removing it can meet extreme resistance and feelings of withdrawal. If you tend towards anxiety, going 'cold turkey' and suddenly avoiding all sugar and stimulants can create a further stress response and profound cravings. Both sugar and caffeine withdrawal produce very real effects, such as headaches, irritability, anger, energy slumps, depression and fatigue. Much of this is a result of interrupted glucose supply to the brain, which causes poor serotonin regulation. Rather than removing sources immediately, supplying quality proteins and fats needed to soothe agitated neurochemistry, and bringing down sympathetic nervous system dominance (via yoga and breath work, for example) can create an environment where sugar can be minimized with least distress. These are discussed more specifically in the next two chapters.

The recipes in this chapter offer support when bringing sugar levels down, to best help stress-coping capacity, alongside reducing sugar cravings and withdrawal.

COFFEE – FRIEND OR FOE?

Coffee can certainly give you a buzz but, like many addictive substances, the initial high is inevitably followed by a low – in effect, a withdrawal symptom. Coffee drinkers often sleep less soundly than non-coffee drinkers, because the caffeine keeps stress hormones up later in the day, when they need to come down to allow good quality sleep via hormones such as melatonin.

You do not necessarily have to give up coffee entirely – just cutting back can help your energy levels to recover. For some people, this may mean cutting down from six daily coffees to one or two; for others, it means going from two to none. If you find this hard, try not to have a coffee or tea before at least 11am, so that you are not relying on a stimulant to kick-start your day. If you do have one first thing, make sure it is after breakfast so that your blood sugar levels are already supported, and the stimulatory effect tempered. As you begin to reduce your intake, you may feel even more tired or headachey; this occurs because the receptors in our brains that pick up and use our energy 'currency' ATP (adenosine tri-phosphate) get accustomed to caffeine taking on that role. When it is removed, they take a few days to resensitize back to utilising your own ATP.

Decaffeinated coffee can be a viable alternative to help wean you off, as it still contains stimulants such as theophylline and threobromine. Choose water-filtered versions to avoid harsh chemicals used to remove caffeine. Black tea is also a good alternative as it has a lot less caffeine, and green tea has only very little, with other soothing properties such as L-theanine (see page 56).

If you follow the guidelines in this book about reducing sugar and caffeine to help boost your energy and maintain even moods, you should find you no longer 'need' so many doses of caffeine.

Key nutrients for calming an anxious mind

Reducing and avoiding sugar and stimulants is best done in a progressive way that still allows you to cope with life, because in this way you will be able to make long-term changes that can stick.

- Balance blood sugar in the morning to support naturally energizing cortisol levels, rather than turning to stress, caffeine and adrenaline to get yourself out of the door.

Making space to eat a supportive breakfast in a calm way can make all the difference to the quality of your day.

• Avoid all stimulants past 4pm, including caffeine, alcohol, sugar and even TV and stimulating factors like screens when you are home from work. Aim for a maximum of two cups of coffee or three cups of tea a day, although for some this might still make you feel agitated. Try to drink these with food to temper their stimulatory effect. Chocolate, cola and some medications also contain caffeine.

• Reduce and then cut out sugar before cutting out caffeine. This is because if you tend to be low on energy and use coffee or tea and sugar to keep going, reducing caffeine will likely increase the sugar cravings. Look at your breakfast and decide if it is helping or hindering you to regulate blood sugar levels, then work towards a gradual decrease in sugar as your tastes adapt to less sweetness.

• Make sure that you have sufficient fats and proteins in your diet to enable the production of neurotransmitters and hormones that get utilized at much higher rates when we are in the heightened mind-body state of stress. We will explore these more in the next two chapters.

FOODS FOR SOOTHING AGITATION

Certain foods and drinks can have a directly soothing effect on the nervous system, taking you out of sympathetic fight-or-flight mode and into a relaxing parasympathetic mode, where we heal, digest and recover but also can begin to quiet a racing mind:

• Drinking relaxing herbal teas has a calming effect as holding mugs or bowls of warm liquids (so soups and stews also work well) have a soothing effect and have even been shown to alleviate feelings of loneliness.

- Chamomile tea is particularly calming as it raises levels of the soothing neurotransmitter glycine long after it has been drunk and even builds this up when taken regularly. If you don't like the taste, try it in a calm or sleep tea formula or add some fresh mint leaves; there are many herb mixes available, too.

- Celery and lettuce contain the chemical apigenin (to a lesser extent) that activates the soothing parasympathetic tone of the nervous system. Celery also contains high levels of the mineral potassium that is needed to bring us down from the stress response, so add it to soups and stews to make particularly reassuring comfort food.

- Licorice tea is a great alternative to coffee or caffeinated black tea as it lifts energy levels but also supports the adrenal glands as an adaptogenic herb (see pages 55–6). Licorice can keep cortisol circulating, though, so don't drink it after 4pm if you have very sensitive sleep and avoid it completely if you have high blood pressure.

Should I take supplements to help me cope with stress?

Ideally we want to be addressing our relationship and responses to the stresses in our life through diet, lifestyle and dealing with the underlying root causes and the habits these lead us to. But while you are exploring this often multi-layered set of circumstances, taking a few key supplements might help you to self-soothe and feel calmer, which will allow you to implement the changes you need to stop yourself giving in to stress-induced cravings and food impulses.

(Also see the considerations in the Sleep Support chapter, pages 214-15.)

Magnesium – the stress-coping, mood-enhancing mineral

There is no more important nutrient to mention in the face of modern stress than magnesium. We need to consume this in large amounts and we use it up quickly in the stress response as it works to create energy (ATP) and get the heart pumping faster and the muscles tightening ready for action. However, it is also needed by the calming parasympathetic nervous system, so if stress depletes our stores, calming down can be difficult and thus we get caught in a state of constant alert. Magnesium deficiency can show up as any symptom relating to nervous system agitation, including anxiety, insomnia, headaches, muscle cramps, PMS, depression, fatigue, fibromyalgia, panic attacks, IBS and blood sugar issues.

It is also needed to produce insulin, so during blood sugar highs and lows, we use up more. In some literature, one molecule of sugar is said to need 56 molecules of magnesium for its metabolism, so eating sugar in excess of our energy needs robs us of this calming mineral.

Optimal magnesium levels are vital if nerve cells (neurones) are to communicate effectively with one another. In the absence of sufficient magnesium, the messages passed between nerve cells using neurotransmitters become excessively 'loud' and can cause more extreme emotional reactions, including moodiness and agitation.

Magnesium may be low in those with mood issues, but also those with digestive, respiratory and muscular conditions. It tends to be poorly ingested in the modern diet, as it is found in green leafy vegetables, nuts, seeds and fish. High-stress lifestyles, emotional stress or personal loss within the last few years may leave us with depleted levels. Magnesium can be depleted by some medications, alcohol use above moderate drinking and exercise over several hours daily.

The UK National Diet and Nutrition Survey (last published, 2016) shows that an average diet provides below 250mg of magnesium per day and the optimal daily intake (food plus supplements) is estimated to be just over 800mg; this is possibly contributing to the rise in mood issues. Modern man tends to get more calcium and less magnesium than our Stone Age counterparts, due to more dairy and fewer green leaves. As these two 'calming minerals' work together (the optimal balance between 2:1 and 1:1 is much discussed), many people benefit from extra magnesium to be able to use both.

Good magnesium food sources in balance with calcium are: green leafy vegetables, nuts, seeds, fish, carrots, sweet potato, avocado, cauliflower, tahini, parsley, soy, whole grains, lentils.

Even if you are having plenty of these foods, but have high stress in your life, feel highly reactive or are suffering from the symptoms mentioned above, it is safe to supplement with extra magnesium.

- Normal magnesium supplementation range: 300–700mg, which can be taken as 300–400mg in the evening to promote sleep, and extra in the morning to help prevent anxiety where needed.
- Best supplement forms are magnesium ascorbate, magnesium citrate or magnesium amino acid chelate.
- Glycine and taurine supplements can help produce sleep neurotransmitters in the evening (see Chapter 7 on Sleep Support).
- Only take calcium or bone-health supplements with magnesium included, ideally with twice as much magnesium as calcium, especially if you eat calcium-rich dairy foods.

Adaptogenic herbs

These herbs work like 'good stress', encouraging resistance and appropriate response to stressors via the brain. They are called adrenal adaptogens as they regulate responses to stress; raising stress hormones when depleted and lowering them when the adrenals are overworking. These herbs include licorice, ginseng, rhodiola, gingko biloba, rhemmania, schisandra and astragalus. Rather than taking each of these substances individually, it is best to find a nutrient-herbal blend that is specifically synergized to have maximum effect.

Buy quality herbal supplements and follow the instructions on the label, building up from the lowest dose. Your healthfood-shop adviser or healthcare practitioner will be able to help you with this, or you can consult a qualified medical herbalist for specific advice.

L-Theanine

L-theanine is a constituent of tea, known to have calming effects on body and mind. Taken in concentrated form in supplements, it may help reduce mental and physical stress and increase mental focus. It is often found in sleep formulas, but can also be taken – like all the supplements in this section – to help promote a calm attitude and body responses throughout the day. They will not make you sleepy, but simply allow your nervous system to come down again after feeling on 'constant alert', where you can feel more clarity, safety and perspective.

As well as the recipes and advice for balancing blood sugar included in Chapter 1, we can offer specific advice for when sugar cravings hit, and also practical ways by which we can look after ourselves when we may be fatigued, demotivated or agitated because of stress.

Supporting the self-soothing capacity of the nervous system helps us to come back down to a calm baseline when we have become reactive or anxious. Many foods provide the nutrients we need to reach both energized and relaxed states, and move between them. When you are choosing your food, ask yourself how close to its natural state it is. The more processed or refined it is, the less likely it is to be rich in the nutrients that nature intended us to have.

High-Five Seeds

Stress can have us feeling less able to nourish ourselves and more likely to snack on sugar or junk fats, so having a quick and satisfying alternative handy when cravings take over can rewire our brains to help us turn to food that supports our resources, rather than depleting them.

Seeds and nuts contain all of the nutrients that satisfy hunger and help us produce energy (except vitamin C), and they can be added to any favourite food, such as a healthy nutty topping for yoghurt, cereal, soups and casseroles. The seeds listed below provide you with a good daily intake of essential fats (see next chapter), as well as calming magnesium, and all in a tasty, versatile form.

You will need to mix together roughly equal amounts of flax, pumpkin, sunflower, sesame and hemp seeds, all of which are available at healthfood shops. These seeds are best eaten well ground, as our teeth can struggle to fully break down such small items. You could use a herb or coffee grinder (kept solely for this purpose, of course, as you won't be able to use it for coffee beans, because of the strong flavours). Seeds contain a high percentage of volatile fats, which are easily damaged by heat and light, so it is important to store the ground mixture in a sealable, airtight jar in the fridge.

Crackers with toppings

Having a healthy savoury snack easily available can help you to wean yourself off a sweet 'treat' habit or even provide an easy breakfast. This is a good choice mid-afternoon if you have a large gap between lunch and dinner.

Choose from oat cakes, rice cakes or rye crackers and top them with:

- Houmous, goat's cheese or smoked salmon with tomatoes, avocado or cucumber.
- Hazelnut or almond butter (you can buy all sorts of tasty nut butters from healthfood shops).
- Smoked fish pâté (see page 124).

Lentils with Spinach

This Iranian dish was traditionally prepared in medieval times to heal the sick. However, it was said that the dish only acted as an effective cure if the ingredients were bought with money that had been begged for in the streets. It is a dense vegan meal or side dish that will support the adrenals and can even be eaten for breakfast, with full-fat plain yoghurt or coconut yoghurt. For those not eating eggs, fish, meat or dairy, pulses can provide protein in the diet, but if you find they create gas or bloating (more common if you are stressed and digestion is struggling, see Chapter 5) cook them in a slow cooker/crockpot or add a stick of kombu seaweed to break down the starches present. This dish freezes well, which means you can always have something nutritious available.

Serves 4

250 g (9 oz) brown lentils

500 g (1 lb 2 oz) fresh spinach or 250 g (9 oz) frozen spinach

½ teaspoon ground coriander

½ teaspoon ground cumin

1 clove garlic, crushed

1 tablespoon olive oil

pinch of salt and freshly ground black pepper

1   Put the lentils into a pan of cold water, bring to the boil and then simmer until they are soft – this should take about an hour.

2   Wash and chop the fresh spinach (or defrost if you're using frozen). Put the spices, garlic and olive oil into a pan with a pinch of salt and pepper over a medium heat. Stir well for a minute before adding the spinach, then stir for a couple more minutes.

3   Drain the lentils, combine with the spinach and either serve immediately or leave to cool before freezing.

Frittata

As we discussed in Chapter 1, eggs are a truly useful food to support blood sugar balance, but they also support the adrenals with their high protein and micro-nutrient content, including the B vitamins discussed in the next chapter. Making a frittata is easy and quick, can be varied to suit your tastes – for instance, by adding any vegetables you like – and can last for several meals, including breakfast and a convenient packed lunch. Here we've included sweet potato as a starchy carbohydrate source for sustained energy that makes you less likely to turn to sugar or stimulants later.

Serves 4

150 g (5 oz) sweet potatoes, cut into chunks

1 tablespoon olive oil

1 red onion, finely sliced

2 courgettes/zucchini, finely sliced

sprig of fresh thyme, leaves picked

6 medium eggs

salt and freshly ground black pepper

1   Put the sweet potatoes into a pan of boiling water and cook for 10–12 minutes until tender. Heat the oil in a large pan and soften the onion for 2–3 minutes without allowing it to brown. Add the courgettes, the thyme, a pinch of salt and some freshly ground black pepper. Cook for another 3 minutes.

2   Stir in the cooked sweet potatoes and remove the pan from the heat. Preheat the grill.

3   Beat the eggs; although you can beat all six eggs together, the fluffiest frittata is made by beating four of the eggs, whole, then whisking the whites of the other two, and folding the whites into the other eggs. Pour the egg mixture over the vegetables in the pan to evenly cover them. Cook on a very low heat for about

8 minutes, until the eggs are nearly set. Place the pan under the grill and cook until the eggs are completely set.

4   Slide the frittata out of the pan onto a plate and, using a fish slice, cut it into generous wedges. You can serve it as it is, warm, or later, cold. Serve with Proper Green Salad (page 321).

Mediterranean Chicken, Egg or Tofu Salad

This basic salad plus protein meal makes a great nutritional mainstay for a lunch or dinner, and if it becomes a real favourite staple you can ring the changes by swapping out the protein part, alternating fish, beans, chicken, egg, tofu, depending on your tastes and eating style. As we will discuss in the next chapter, protein provides the building blocks for mental health, and also helps us cope with stress via blood sugar balance. The green leaves are a must, as they provide a host of minerals, including magnesium, and so they can be extra calming, particularly if you use lettuce (see page 53).

Serves 2

3–4 large handfuls of cos lettuce, washed baby spinach, watercress, rocket or other green salad

4 spring onions/scallions, finely chopped

8 cherry tomatoes, quartered

2 cold grilled/broiled chicken breasts, 2 boiled eggs or 200 g (7 oz) marinated tofu chunks

For the dressing

2 dessertspoons extra virgin olive oil

4 basil leaves, torn or chopped

1 teaspoon wholegrain mustard

1 dessertspoon balsamic vinegar

freshly ground black pepper

1   Arrange half of the salad ingredients on each plate and place your
    chosen protein on top.

2   Put the dressing ingredients in a jar, screw on the lid and shake
    well. Pour the dressing over the salad just before serving.

3   For an oriental spin, use the Oriental Bite dressing (see page 31),
    or for a delicious French twist, use the Tangy Vinaigrette
    (see page 31).

Roasted Sweet Vegetables

Including sweet tastes in the vegetable part of your meals can make them more enticing when you feel the urge for fast food, and it also provides some ready brain-energy when you're feeling drained. This dish can also be used as an alternative to starchy grains if they do not agree with your digestion or worsen your blood sugar issues.

The sweet potato, squash and beetroot/beet make a good starch part of any meal, even a hastily prepared supper, as they cook relatively quickly, but if only two out of the three ingredients are available, it's fine to just include those. This is also great as a snack or small meal in a bowl, with seeds, feta or houmous for added taste and texture.

When you are buying sweet potatoes, go for the ones with the orange flesh rather than the white, as they are sweeter. You can always make double the quantity given here if you want leftovers for lunch the next day to eat cold with a salad.

Serves 4

1 large sweet potato, sliced into
  1 cm (½ inch) rounds
½ butternut squash/pumpkin,
  sliced into 1 cm (½ inch)
  rounds

2 fresh beetroot/beet, cut into
  1 cm (½ inch) slices
extra virgin olive oil, for drizzling
freshly ground black pepper

1   Preheat the oven to 190°C/375°F/Gas Mark 5.
2   Place all the prepared vegetables in a baking pan (ideally lined
    with baking paper to prevent them sticking and make washing up
    easier!). Drizzle olive oil all over the top and season with freshly
    ground black pepper. Bake in the oven until cooked – this should
    take 20–30 minutes. Prick a few of the vegetables with a skewer
    to check that they are soft before serving.

Red Cabbage and Feta Salad

The sharp taste and crunchy texture of red cabbage go beautifully with a rich feta cheese, providing satisfaction to a stressed mind and body on both counts. The red cabbage provides bulk to satisfy the appetite and sulphur compounds that aid detoxification – cleansing processes that need to work harder in the face of stress. You can also add a diced apple to this dish, which will provide another texture, and the sweetness of the apple blends well with the other flavours while also sating any sweet craving the brain might be seeking because of long-term stress.

Serves 2

½ large red cabbage, finely shredded

150 g (5 oz) feta cheese, crumbled

1 apple, diced (optional)

2 tablespoons sunflower seeds

4 tablespoons Tangy Vinaigrette (see page 31)

1 Mix the shredded cabbage with the crumbled cheese, chopped apple (if you're using it) and sunflower seeds. Toss well in the vinaigrette just before serving.

Fruit Whizz

These delicious refreshing desserts are super fast to make and provide a sweet yet healthy choice for anyone craving sugar or struggling to go without a habitual dessert after a meal, helping you enjoy a little sweet taste that's not too sugary. They can be frozen in lolly moulds for ice-cream alternatives in summer, too.

The two recipes here represent variations on the same theme – one with summer berries and one with tropical fruits – and each has a completely different taste. The Summer Whizz, because of the hot fruit sauce, is actually lovely in the winter, too, just replace the fresh summer fruits with frozen.

Summer Whizz
Serves 4

500 g (1 lb 2 oz) fresh or frozen summer fruits
100 g (3½ oz) plain yoghurt
½ teaspoon vanilla essence

2 teaspoons clear honey
2 tablespoons kirsch or red wine (optional, for a more 'sophisticated' dessert)

1 Put half of the fruit in a blender with the yoghurt and the vanilla and blend until smooth. Pour the mixture into a freezerproof container with a lid and put it into the freezer for at least 1 hour. Remove and stir it a couple of times during the hour to stop it crystallizing too much.

2 When the fruit whizz is almost frozen, put the rest of the fruit in a saucepan with the honey and the kirsch or wine (if using) over a low heat, gently bring to the boil and cook for a minute or so. If the mixture is particularly watery, simmer until it has reduced a bit.

3   Scoop the frozen whizz into bowls and pour the hot fruit sauce over the top, then serve immediately.

Tropical Whizz
Serves 4

250 g (9 oz) bag frozen tropical fruit

100 g (3½ oz) plain yoghurt

1 tablespoon desiccated/dried shredded coconut

2 tablespoons pineapple juice

2 teaspoons good-quality honey (optional, wean off to none)

4 slices fresh pineapple

2 passionfruits

1   Put the tropical fruit in a blender with the yoghurt, coconut and pineapple juice and blend until it is completely smooth. Pour the mixture into a freezerproof container with a lid and put it into the freezer for at least 1 hour. Remove and stir it a couple of times during the hour to stop it crystallizing too much.

2   When the fruit whizz is almost frozen, drizzle the honey over the pineapple slices, put them into a hot griddle pan and cook for 1–2 minutes on each side until they start to turn slightly brown.

3   Put a pineapple slice on each plate and top with a scoop of the whizz. Slice the passionfruits in half and scoop the contents of each half on top of the whizz. Serve immediately.

Chocolate Pudding

This delight is remarkably unwicked for such a luxurious result, especially when you consider that research has shown that 40 g (1½ oz) a day of plain/bittersweet chocolate helps people cope with stress! Plain/bittersweet chocolate is rich in anti-inflammatory and heart-protective polyphenol antioxidants that are also found in wine and green tea. Remember, though, chocolate is bitter so when you buy it it will always have some form of sugar added. Don't be fooled by talk of 'natural sugars', if it's sweet it contains sugar in some form, so choose small amounts of high-quality chocolate with a high cocoa solid percentage (70 per cent and above). In this way you take advantage of the 'happy chemical' beta endorphins – but don't kid yourself, much of this effect comes from the combination of sugar and fat – and PEA (the 'love molecule') which it contains.

You can vary this dish by adding a little orange juice or mint essence.

Serves 4

600 ml (1 pint) almond or coconut milk

75–100 g (2½–3½ oz) plain/bittersweet organic chocolate (at least 70% cocoa solids)

4 medium eggs or 1 whole avocado

¼ teaspoon salt

1 teaspoon vanilla essence

1   Preheat the oven to 170°C/325°F/Gas Mark 3.

2   Put the milk and chocolate into a saucepan over a low heat, stirring gently until the chocolate is melted and well mixed in with the milk. Do not allow it to boil. Remove from the heat and leave to cool.

3   Put the eggs or avocado, salt and vanilla into a blender and slowly add the cooled chocolatey milk until it is all well blended. Pour the mixture into 4 individual ovenproof dishes and bake in the oven for 40 minutes or until set.

4   These puddings can be served hot or cold – once cool, cover them with cling film/plastic wrap and keep in the fridge until you are ready to serve.

Which lifestyle changes will help you cope with stress?

How we live determines the quality of our days, and noticing when the heart-racing, blood-pumping, tight-jawed feelings of stress emerge can help you to navigate through life with more ease. This has a far-reaching effect on blood sugar and cravings, in turn helping to bring down stress levels and impact other related health issues, including weight gain.

Exercise – but not too much

Exercise also plays a part in restoring the health of the adrenals, but not in the way you might expect. Many people who have fast-paced lives that exhaust their adrenals also follow a very rigorous exercise routine, not realizing that this too acts as a stressor. When you are run down, doing a hard workout at the gym is actually the last thing you need. Exercise increases levels of adrenaline, cortisol and the 'happy chemicals' beta-endorphins, which is partly why, when you have just finished the workout or run, you may feel particularly good. However, if you are suffering from adrenal burnout, too much exercise only exacerbates the problem.

So if you are experiencing stress symptoms, it is far better to do more moderate exercise – for example, walking, gentle swimming, yoga or a walk-run combination – that engages your whole body and increases circulation, while only slightly increasing your heart rate.

Walking away

Walking is our most natural form of exercise and helps stress hormones to lower as the movement loosens tight tissues and helps the shoulders and jaw to release. These parts of the body often become tense with stress, so relaxing them lets your whole mind-body know that it can come down from these heightened responses. Stress can be exacerbated when we sit at a desk all day and then only move suddenly at the gym or when we go for a run – it's quite a shock to the system! Instead, we need to move regularly – getting up and stretching, moving freely and taking a walk break can help relieve stress accumulation throughout the day.

Talk it out

No dietary changes will restore your adrenal function to a normal level if you do not tackle any external sources of stress. This may involve reassessing your work, home or social life. If the stress is ongoing and you reach the stage where you feel you cannot cope, it is important to seek support. Talk to a sympathetic partner, friend, relative or colleague, or enlist the help of a life coach or professional counsellor (see pages 281–2).

TOP TIPS FOR CALMING AN ANXIOUS MIND

- See the blood sugar supporting recommendations in Chapter I and the tips on page 40.
- Prioritize having breakfast every day and allow yourself the time to pause and start the day from a calm place.
- Examine your relationship with 'stimulants' such as sugar and sugary foods or drinks, refined foods (including biscuits or white bread), coffee, tea, alcohol and cigarettes. Bring down your level of consumption of these at a balanced rate so that your body and brain can get used to the change. Reduce the sweet ingredients in your diet, too, and use starchy vegetables to provide energy.
- Allow yourself 1–2 cups a day of caffeinated drinks, replacing these with calming herbal teas for the rest of the day.
- Take nutrients designed to support your adrenal glands, especially magnesium, if needed.
- At least three times a week, take moderate exercise, such as walking, gentle swimming, or yoga.
- Get up from your desk and make sure you move about regularly throughout the day.
- Walk regularly, and as often as possible try to do so in fresh air and nature.
- Take steps to reduce any stressful issues in your life, ideally calling on someone else who can help.

Part Three

RECIPES FOR SUPPORTING BRAIN FOCUS

CHAPTER 3

FOCUS AND CONCENTRATION SUPPORT

From the foundations of blood sugar balance and stress support that we now have discussed, we can add in some specific nutritional help for the workings of our brains. Providing constant energy from a steady supply of slow-release sugars and reducing stress hormones to help mind clarity and attention are crucial for us to be able to focus and maintain concentration, but we can also improve other aspects of brain function through food.

For optimal mental health and cognitive function we need healthy nerves and optimal levels of neurotransmitters (brain messenger molecules), and these need a plentiful supply of nutrients to work. Indeed, pretty much all the systems in our body need to be in good working order, even those governing our digestion and detoxification (see Chapter 5). And without an optimal nutrient supply, these systems will still work, but they may not function as well as they should. For example, we know that a deficiency in vitamin C causes scurvy, characterized by cracks at the corners of the mouth and mouth ulcers. Although such severe vitamin deficiencies are now rare in developed countries, research has shown that even slightly reduced nutrient levels are clearly linked to a decline in brain function and mood.

On the list below, tick the symptoms that are familiar and persistent for you:

- Lowered ability to stick to one task.
- Memory not what it used to be.
- Brain fog, particularly in the afternoon.
- Deteriorating memory.
- Difficulty sustaining concentration.
- Feeling tired all the time.
- Using coffee, tea or a cigarette to get you going in the morning.
- Feeling unrefreshed after sleep.
- Experiencing energy slumps during the day.
- Having mood and concentration swings.
- Craving sweet and starchy foods, coffee, tea, alcohol, cigarettes.
- Getting angry easily.
- Over-reacting to pressing or antagonistic issues.
- Regularly feeling impatient.
- Feeling anxious or nervous.

If you ticked five or more symptoms, this is a sign you need to pay attention to your mind-body and to make sure you include quality food sources in your diet, covering the building blocks that your brain needs. Although the list of symptoms that can result from even a mild nutrient deficiency is seemingly endless, mood swings, irritability, tiredness and poor concentration are all classic signs that your brain, and the rest of your body, are not receiving all the nutrients they need.

Why do I feel this way?

Every single process and chemical reaction that takes place in your body depends on a regular supply of micro nutrients, such as vitamins and minerals, as well as macro nutrients, protein, carbohydrates, fats and water, which we need in larger amounts. It makes sense, then, that the raw materials you feed your body affect the way it works and have an impact on your moods and energy levels. We need to produce neurotransmitters (brain chemicals) for all our moods and to sustain focused attention; so in this chapter we look more generally at the building blocks of our diet that we need for optimal brain function, particularly key nutrients such as quality proteins and B vitamins.

Serotonin and dopamine – focus, concentration and mood

Biochemically, mood state is very much dependent on having enough of two particular neurotransmitters (brain-messenger molecules): serotonin and dopamine. When levels of these are low, a similar mood is likely to follow, leaving you ill-equipped to cope with stress. In fact, many common anti-depressant drugs are designed to increase levels of serotonin and dopamine: the most commonly prescribed SSRIs (selective serotonin reuptake inhibitor) keep serotonin from being reabsorbed by the nerve cells, therefore increasing its availibility.

In stressed states we produce more of the motivating, excitatory neurotransmitters to keep us alert and responsive. This means that when stress is chronic and ongoing, their levels become depleted over time, in part because we are struggling to produce enough to keep up with demand, and in part because the receptor sites that pick these up to be used in the brain can become desensitized – they just don't 'see' them anymore.

People with low dopamine and/or serotonin levels often get more of a kick from stimulating or numbing substances such as sugar, alcohol, junk food, recreational drugs and addictive medications such as benzodiazepines (a member of the highly addictive Valium family). High stress helps to make these substances habit-forming. We might have a sudden rise of these feelgood brain chemicals (and 'happy' beta-endorphins, too), but they then cause crashes later, leading to cycles of dependence and an increasing reliance on them to 'feel normal' and be able to focus and concentrate, let alone maintain a chirpy mood.

Stress also uses up all of the nutrients we need not only to create these neurotransmitters, but also to produce healthy neurons – the nerve cells that transmit electrical nerve impulses all through our nervous system, which is how our brain and body communicate at all times. Healthy fats are needed for this transmission and to pick up and use the neurotransmitters, and we'll focus on their role in mood maintenance in the next chapter.

Bare essentials for focusing our minds

Here is a breakdown of the nutrients needed for producing and using serotonin and dopamine. All of these are gobbled up by stress as they are also needed to produce energy, as well as the cascade of hormones, enzymes and other neurotransmitters that we produce in this reactive state.

For a list of foods that are rich in many of the nutrients mentioned here, see the chart opposite.

	Role	Nutrients needed
Serotonin	Feel-good neurotransmitter. Needed for good moods, healthy sleep patterns and appetite control	Vitamins B3, B6, biotin, folic acid, tryptophan (see below), zinc
Dopamine	Stimulating neurotransmitter. Needed for feeling motivation and pleasure	Vitamins B3, B6, B12, C, folic acid, copper, iron, magnesium (see p.54), manganese, phenylalanine, tyrosine (see p.82), zinc
Healthy neurons	Nerve cells required for general health and to transmit messages efficiently	Antioxidants (see p.116), B vitamins, essential fatty acids (see Chapter 4), folic acid, magnesium
Even blood sugar levels (see Chapter 1)	Dives in blood sugar send mood, energy and concentration crashing	B vitamins, chromium, magnesium, vanadium, zinc

Tryptophan for serotonin production

You can help to eat yourself happy by eating foods rich in the amino acid (protein building block) tryptophan, which is a precursor to the mood-boosting neurotransmitter serotonin. Considerable quantities of tryptophan are found in chicken, turkey, red meat, tofu, legumes, lentils, oats, fish, eggs, bananas, figs, milk, cheese, seaweed, sunflower seeds and yoghurt. However, you need to be aware that eating large amounts of these foods (apart from being somewhat repetitive) is not guaranteed to ensure that the tryptophan they contain will actually be converted into serotonin in the brain.

For a start, tryptophan can also be transformed into other substances once it has been absorbed into your system. Also, you need a good supply of certain nutrients – such as vitamins B3, B6, C and folic acid, biotin and zinc – for the conversion into serotonin to take place. There is also another potential drawback, too: when you eat foods that contain other amino acids (that is most protein-rich foods), they tend to beat tryptophan to the transport vehicles that carry it across into the brain, leaving your serotonin raw material on the outside. However, eating foods rich in carbohydrates, even if they do not contain tryptophan themselves, helps increase the amount of tryptophan from other foods that is actually transported across into the brain, as there is less competition for the carriers. This is probably why many people crave starchy or sweet foods when they are feeling down – to raise serotonin levels – and we'll explore how to help this.

To increase your levels of tryptophan, and thus serotonin, try to include some of the tryptophan-rich foods listed above in your daily diet. Also, notice when you may need to include unrefined, wholesome, carbohydrate-rich foods, such as brown rice or wholegrain bread, and follow the advice in Chapter 6 on appetite regulation. In addition, take a multivitamin/ mineral supplement (see page 278) to make sure you are covering the whole spectrum of nutrients that you need on a daily basis.

Tyrosine for dopamine and stress management

Tyrosine is an amino acid that is needed to produce dopamine, but it is also important for adrenal function and how we cope with stress. It is found in almonds, avocados, bananas, dairy products, butter/lima beans, pumpkin seeds and sesame seeds. Dopamine promotes alertness, mood, motivation and activity, so eating these tyrosine-rich foods can help prevent us turning to stimulants such as caffeine and refined sugars that upset blood sugar balance. Sugar should be avoided because it provokes a 'dopamine response', lighting up the reward centres in our brains and giving us an immediate mood lift, but in reality this is not the lifting of a clear, sustained mood, but rather a drug-like effect that has us coming back for more.

Active ingredient: B vitamins

Inside each cell in the body are minute energy factories called mitochondria. How much brain energy and focus you have relies on the production of energy inside every single one of these microscopic powerhouses. For energy to be created, a combustion process takes place, and to fuel this the mitochondria require a constant supply of glucose, oxygen and nutrients. Among the key nutrient players here are vitamins B1, B3, B5, B6 and biotin (another B vitamin). B vitamins are also needed to help maintain healthy nerves and to produce the important neurotransmitters (there are plenty more on top of serotonin and dopamine!) that help maintain concentration, mood and control appetite.

The B vitamins' role may also be linked to the way in which they keep nerves healthy and help the production of substances called phospholipids – such as phosphatidyl choline (see box, page 86) and phosphatidyl serine – that combine with essential fatty acids (see next chapter) to make cell membranes.

Deficiencies in certain nutrients, particularly some of the B vitamins, are clearly associated with depression. In fact, a deficiency in most of the B vitamins is linked to some sort of decline in mental or emotional state: depression, fatigue, confusion, memory loss, apathy, anxiety, irritability, nervousness, sleep disturbances, sluggishness or loss of appetite. Vitamin B1 (thiamine) was originally known as the nerve vitamin because its deficiency causes beri beri, a nerve disease. A severe deficiency of vitamin B3 (niacin) is called pellagra – as well as skin redness and digestive problems, symptoms of this condition include fatigue, insomnia, apathy and even manic depression. Folic acid, another member of the B-vitamin family, is believed to be the most commonly deficient nutrient in the world – recent UK government research found that more than half of girls in their late teens were getting less than the recommended amount of folic acid from their diet. The most common symptom of a folic-acid deficiency is depression.

When we are under stress, we tend to eat a diet high in refined foods, which have been depleted of the B vitamins and other nutrients nature provided them with. For example, refined flour contains less than a quarter of the level of vitamin B1 and a fifth of the B3 found in its wholegrain counterpart. You should also try to steer clear of the substances that hamper the absorption and use of some B vitamins in the body – alcohol, caffeine and some drugs, including the contraceptive pill, are all culprits.

So, although the demand for B vitamins is higher, we are not necessarily meeting this increased need.

That's why it is so important to include plenty of foods that are rich in B vitamins in your diet, including sunflower seeds, nuts, mushrooms, eggs, fish, lean meat and poultry (see below).

In addition to eating a diet rich in fresh, whole foods and avoiding refined foods, taking a B-complex vitamin supplement (or a multivitamin and mineral supplement that is high in B vitamins) can help ensure that you are getting enough of these important nutrients. Do remember, though, that supplements are not a substitute for eating well, cutting out stimulants and getting enough sleep.

Best B-vitamin food sources

You'll note from this list that many of the top sources of B vitamins are not vegan, so if you eat little or no animal produce, make sure you have plenty of the plant sources, as the levels of protein and B vitamins, and other focus and mood nutrients (such as magnesium, iron and zinc), are less concentrated in plant foods. Vegans who are stressed, tired or find it hard to concentrate should definitely consider taking a multivitamin and mineral with good levels of B vitamins.

Vitamin B1
Beef kidney and liver, brewer's yeast, brown rice, chickpeas, kidney beans, pork, rice bran, salmon, soy beans, sunflower seeds, wheatgerm, wholegrain wheat and rye.

Vitamin B2
Almonds, brewer's yeast, cheese, chicken, mushrooms, wheatgerm.

Vitamin B3
Beef liver, brewer's yeast, chicken, eggs, fish, sunflower seeds, turkey.

Vitamin B5
Blue cheese, brewer's yeast, corn, eggs, lentils, liver, lobster, meats, peanuts, peas, soy beans, sunflower seeds, wheatgerm.

Vitamin B6
Avocados, bananas, bran, brewer's yeast, carrots, hazelnuts, lentils, rice, salmon, shrimps, soy beans, sunflower seeds, tuna, walnuts, wheatgerm, wholegrain flour.

B-vitamin-compatible nutrients for brain energy production
Protein
Dairy products, eggs, fish, meat, poultry, soy beansm pulses, nuts and seeds, quinoa.

Vitamin C
Blackcurrants, broccoli, Brussels sprouts, cabbage, grapefruit,

green peppers, guava, kale, lemons, oranges, papaya, potatoes, spinach, strawberries, tomatoes, watercress.

Magnesium
Almonds, fish, green leafy vegetables, kelp, molasses, nuts, soy beans, sunflower seeds, wheatgerm.

Zinc
Egg yolks, fish, all meat, milk, molasses, oysters, sesame seeds, soy beans, sunflower seeds, turkey, wheatgerm, whole grains.

Chromium
Beef, brewer's yeast, chicken, eggs, fish, fruit, milk products, potatoes, whole grains.

Coenzyme Q10
All foods, particularly beef, mackerel, sardines, soy oil, spinach.

FOCUS ON CHOLINE

Choline, which is a member of the B-vitamin family, has two major functions in the body associated with memory and the brain: it is needed for the structure of brain cells and also to make one of the key messaging neurotransmitters.

Provided there is a good supply of all the B vitamins and other nutrients, the body uses choline to produce phosphatidylcholine, which is incorporated into the membrane of each brain cell. Healthy membranes are, of course, vital if messages such as those that trigger memory are to be transmitted efficiently.

The transmission of memory messages also depends on the body's supply of acetylcholine, the main neurotransmitter responsible for memory and cognitive thinking. The body produces acetylcholine from choline. Some scientists have shown that a lack of choline can result in neurons cannibalizing their own membranes for the choline needed to make acetylcholine.

Although the human body can make small amounts of choline in the liver, this is usually not enough to maintain healthy brain cells, so we need a regular intake of choline through our diet. Many foods contain choline (or at least phosphatidylcholine). Particularly rich sources are cauliflower, eggs, fish, liver, milk and legumes (such as peanuts and soy beans). A large egg is likely to contain 200–300mg of choline. In a study of healthy elderly people, those given 500mg of choline a day performed better in memory tests and reported fewer memory lapses than those not taking it. If you are eating a varied diet that includes some of the foods mentioned above, you are probably providing your body with the generally recommended intake of 500mg a day.

Lecithin, which is a substance derived from eggs or soy, contains about 20 per cent phosphatidylcholine and about 13 per cent choline, although some brands are specially formulated to contain more. You can sprinkle lecithin powder on cereal or soups to increase your daily choline intake.

Just like the recipes in the last two chapters, these provide good levels of the various nutrients needed for brain focus and concentration, as well as a good mood. We need a variety of foods and combinations to cover all of the nutrients and to meet our changing needs at different times, so here we focus on quality proteins that provide good levels of the amino acids we need in constant supply for good mood throughout the day.

Buckwheat Crepes

This is a variation on the traditional French *galettes de sarrasin*, deliciously light pancakes that use buckwheat flour instead of wheat to provide wholegrain energy without the potentially inflammatory effects of wheat (see page 180). Eggs are the perfect foodstuff; rich in protein, B vitamins and also zinc and iron that all work with these for brain function.

For vegans, one mashed banana can replace one egg in cakes and pancakes, but while bananas do provide some tryptophan, they lack the protein of eggs. You can buy pre-prepared egg replacements, but they are often simply starchy tapioca and flour-based, so search for seaweed-('algal') based ones for more protein.

You can serve these with pretty much anything you fancy, such as plain yoghurt, blueberries or apple compote, or use them as the base for a savoury breakfast of scrambled eggs, vegetarian sausages and baked beans, or wilted spinach and crumbled goat's cheese. They can also be used as wraps in place of bread products and freeze well to be used later.

Serves 2

100 g (3½ oz) buckwheat flour
pinch of salt
150 ml (5 fl oz) milk, almond or
    hemp milk

150 ml (5 fl oz) water
1 egg
olive oil, for frying

1   Put the flour and salt into a mixing bowl. Mix the milk and water together in a jug. Beat the egg into the flour, adding the milk and water a little at a time to make a batter. Set aside at room temperature for at least 1 hour.

2   Lightly oil a frying pan and place it over a medium heat. Put a tablespoon of batter into the pan and roll it around to cover the base, right to the edges. Cook it until the pancake is golden, about 2 minutes, then turn it over to cook the other side.

3   Serve hot with your choice of topping.

Mushroom Pâté

Pâtés are easy to whip up and are great to have on hand as a brain booster. This is a dense source of texture, flavours and nutrients to help fuel your focus and stop you turning to less satisfying and sweeter snacks. You can vary the herbs to suit your tastes and experiment with the different components according to your preferences.

As discussed on page 152, mushrooms support gut health which is so important for mood and brain function, but are also important, nutrient-dense sources for those following a plant-based diet.

Serves 2 as lunch, or 4 as a starter

4 medium chestnut mushrooms, trimmed

2 spring onions/scallions, roughly chopped

1 cooked chicken breast, shredded or 200 g (7 oz) cashews for a vegan version

50 g (2 oz) soft goat's or cottage cheese, or vegan 'cheese', crumbled

2 tablespoons olive oil

1 teaspoon chopped tarragon, plus extra to garnish (optional)

1 teaspoon chopped parsley, plus extra to garnish (optional)

pinch of salt and freshly ground black pepper

1   Put the mushrooms, spring onions and chicken or cashews in a blender with all the other ingredients. For a rougher pâté, simply chop the chicken/cashews, mushrooms and spring onions very finely and mix all the ingredients in a bowl. Cover and put in the fridge to chill. If the pâté is for a dinner party, you can transfer it to four individual ramekins.

2   Before serving, garnish with fresh tarragon or parsley. Eat with rye or rice crackers or crudités as a starter or with a large salad as a meal in itself.

Versatile Rice Salad

Rice can make a great base for salads that can be eaten as snacks, whole meals or side dishes. If you choose the 'brown' version, the grain still has its hull intact, meaning that you eat the soluble fibre, B vitamins and zinc found there, as well as the starchy inner 'white' part. Basmati rice is known to release its sugars slower than short-grained types, and wild rice has more immune-protecting antioxidants.

You can load this salad up with any form of protein that suits you, and if you're vegan or simply enjoy the taste and crunch, add some extra seeds or nuts.

This, like any food, can even be eaten for breakfast – we've just become conditioned to believing that only certain foods are 'breakfast foods' thanks to the Victorians, who loved such categorizations. This is particularly good if you want to make a meal in the evening and leave some for breakfast the next day, or if you exercise early and need something to replenish protein and energy stores immediately after. A rice-based salad also freezes well, so you can take a frozen portion to work, where it can defrost during the morning and remain refrigerated for your lunch – the perfect convenience meal!

Note: It is important to be aware that uncooked rice contains spores of the bacteria *Bacillus cereus* that can survive the cooking process. If rice is cooled slowly – left between 5°C and 60°C for too long – they can grow and produce a toxin that causes food poisoning. So just cook as much as you need at the time, or refrigerate (or freeze) very quickly to below 5°C.

Serves 2–3

200 g (7 oz) brown rice (basmati if possible), or a combination of brown and wild rice

3 eggs (vegans can use 150 g/ 5 oz marinated tofu)

1 green pepper, deseeded and finely chopped

4 spring onions/scallions, finely sliced

12 olives, pitted and roughly chopped

8 mint leaves, roughly chopped

1 × 200 g (7 oz) smoked mackerel or salmon fillet (optional)

1 heaped tablespoon capers

3 tablespoons olive oil

juice of ½ lemon

3 large tomatoes, peeled, deseeded and roughly chopped

pinch of salt and freshly ground black pepper

1 Cook the rice following the packet instructions and set aside to cool. Cook the eggs in a pan of boiling water for 9 minutes until they are hard-boiled. Drain and leave until cool enough to handle.

2 Add the vegetables, mint, mackerel or salmon, if using, and all the other ingredients except the tomatoes to the cooled rice and toss the whole mixture well. Add the tomatoes just before eating. If you don't think you're going to eat all the salad in one sitting, just add the tomatoes to individual plates, as they are likely to 'turn' before the rest of the ingredients do.

Spiced Bean Stew

Beans and pulses are an important part of a vegan and vegetarian diet as they are high in protein, but they are also a great starch alternative for everyone. This recipe is for a fast version of the traditionally slow-cooked stew, but if you prefer, you can simply put all the ingredients into a slow cooker (crockpot) to increase digestibility – especially if beans make you gassy, as this can affect brain clarity.

The spices here are known to support circulation and protect neurons, as well as helping balance blood sugar, so this blend can be used as a blueprint for any brain-supporting soup or stew. For extra heat for circulation, ginger can also be added and you can spice up the beans further by adding a dash of chilli powder, which can really wake the brain up!

Serves 3–4

1 onion, chopped
2 cloves garlic, crushed
1 dessertspoon olive oil
1 teaspoon ground cumin
½ teaspoon ground cardamom
½ teaspoon paprika
½ teaspoon ground cinnamon

3 large tomatoes, peeled and chopped
2 x 420 g (15 oz) cans mixed beans, drained
chopped parsley, to garnish
plain yoghurt or coconut yoghurt, to serve

1   Soften the onion and garlic in a large pan with the olive oil. Add the spices and stir well for a few minutes. Add in the tomatoes and then the beans, pouring in a can of water at the same time, and leave the mixture to simmer for at least 30 minutes over a low heat until the beans have softened and the stew has thickened.

2   Serve the stew garnished with a generous amount of chopped parsley and a dollop of yoghurt.

Thai-style Fish

With such emphasis on oily fish for omega 3 levels (see next chapter), white fish can be overlooked as the less healthy version, but for those who eat fish it provides another protein-packed and nutrient-dense alternative that picks up flavours well. Be sure to source sustainable varieties, though; read labels for advice from organizations like the Marine Conservation Society and check for logos from verifying bodies such as the Marine Stewardship Council (MSC). You can use any white fish for this dish, but Atlantic cod and haddock (not line-caught) are the most sustainable and work well. The zestiness of this dish wakes up the brain naturally and goes well with a simple salad of plenty of green leaves for minerals, such as magnesium for focus and concentration.

Serves 4

2½ cm (1 inch) piece of fresh ginger root

2 cloves garlic

1 lime

1 dessertspoon tamari or soy sauce

3–4 dashes of Tabasco sauce

4 white fish steaks, skinned

1   Grate the ginger, garlic and the lime zest into an ovenproof baking dish. Squeeze in the juice of the lime, along with the tamari or soy sauce and Tabasco sauce and stir well.

2   Place the fish steaks in the dish and coat with the marinade. Ideally, marinate the fish for a couple of hours.

3   Preheat the oven to 200°C/400°F/Gas Mark 6. Add 4 tablespoons of water to the fish and mix with the marinade before putting the dish into the oven. Bake for 20 minutes, until cooked through – the flesh should be opaque when you cut it.

4   Serve with steamed or stir-fried vegetables, brown rice or Roasted Sweet Vegetables (see page 64).

Som Tam
(Green Papaya Salad)

Traditionally from the Isaan region of northeastern Thailand, this dish is made freshly to order with a mortar and pestle at street stalls and served with sticky rice and grilled chicken. This is a som tam farang – foreigner's som tam – minus the copious chillies, pungent dried prawns and whole, pickled raw crab! It's best to visit your local Asian grocer to stock up on the ingredients. The papaya is great for digestion, which you'll see is so important for brain function in Chapter 4, but if you can't get hold of it, use half a white cabbage instead.

The authentic Thai version features peanuts rather than cashews, but we've swapped these out as peanuts are a legume rather than a nut, so you lose out on all of the essential oils (see next chapter).

You can add any extra protein in the form of tofu, sliced boiled eggs, prawns or any fish or meat if you are not vegan or vegetarian.

Serves 4

1 clove garlic

1 bird's-eye chilli

1 dessertspoon coconut palm sugar (jageree from Indian grocers)

2 tablespoons roasted cashew nuts

10 runner beans, roughly chopped

4 cherry tomatoes

½ green papaya, finely shredded

juice of 2 limes

1 dessertspoon tamarind concentrate, diluted with same amount of water

1 tablespoon fish sauce

1   In a mortar, crush the garlic, chilli, coconut palm sugar and cashew nuts. Add the runner beans and tomatoes, pounding all the time.

2   Little by little, add the shredded papaya, continuing to pound. Slowly add the lime juice, the tamarind juice and fish sauce, continuing to pound. Taste to see whether you prefer it a little sharper (with a little more lime and tamarind) or saltier (with a little more fish sauce).

3   Serve immediately.

Khosaf

There are times when we simply have to keep going even though we can feel our energy is flagging and our concentration is fading. This is often at the naturally low blood sugar time of around 4pm, which is when you may find yourself most susceptible to raiding the biscuit tin. Having a smart snack on hand that provides the sweetness your brain is crying out for but doesn't worsen the issue, can help alleviate a nagging craving. This Middle Eastern staple makes a filling dessert or a good afternoon snack. The nuts provide the protein, B vitamins, magnesium, zinc and essential oils your brain needs to stay focused. You can increase the nut content and decrease the quantity of dried fruits as your need for sweet tastes reduces.

This recipe serves 6, so you can reduce the quantities if you want to feed fewer people, or store the leftovers in the fridge to eat over a few days. You can also change this up by experimenting with other dried fruits, such as figs or peaches. You should be able to find rose or orange blossom water at a Middle Eastern grocer or in the baking section of a good supermarket, but you can just use water if you can't get either.

Serves 6

1 tablespoon good-quality honey

250 g (10 oz) dried apricots
(unsulphured if possible)

150 g (5 oz) prunes

100 g (3½ oz) almonds

100 g (3½ oz) pine nuts or
sunflower seeds

2 tablespoons rose or orange
blossom water (or 1
tablespoon of each)

1   In a large bowl, melt the honey in half a mug of boiling water.
Add the dried fruits, nuts and seeds, if using, and cover with cold
water. Pour in the rose and/or orange blossom water and mix
well. Leave in the fridge for at least 48 hours for the flavours
to infuse.

2   Serve the Khosaf as it is or with vanilla yoghurt (see page 38).

Which lifestyle changes best support your focus and concentration?

As well as following the stress-reducing advice given on pages 71-2, observing how you make your way through the day can spare the nutrients that would otherwise be used to produce energy to deal with a high-stress reaction. We have finite energy and we need regular periods of recovery and downtime for our minds to be able to fully focus; simply keeping going is a false economy – you wouldn't expect your mobile phone to keep working if you didn't recharge it.

The importance of breath

Our most useful guide to what's happening in our nervous system is the breath. If you just keep going on with high expectations, pushing past your limits, you may notice that your breath becomes quicker and shallower in an attempt to keep energy levels and alertness up. This is unsustainable in the long term as it creates an imbalance of oxygen coming in as you inhale, with carbon dioxide being released as you exhale.

Focusing on long, slow out-breaths can help calm the whole of our mind and body from a racing state, allow us to come back to a place where we can be present and focused, and help us to have perspective and the ability to see the long-term picture. This quality of sustainable attention is known as 'coherence'.

Taking breaks

Becoming aware of when you are about to become overwhelmed and being able to back away can be the difference between collapsing at the end of the day – and avoiding burnout – and actually being more productive and enjoying life because we benefit from a period of not being under pressure. Put breaks into your diary to improve your productivity at work, preferably getting up and moving or taking a walk, to reduce stress hormones and increase blood circulation to the brain.

A word on sleep

Getting a night of good-quality sleep is fundamental to optimal cognitive ability and focus during the day – see Chapter 7 for more help for brain recovery in dreamland.

TOP TIPS FOR FOCUS AND CONCENTRATION

Add the following measures to the blood-sugar-balancing and stress-coping foundations from Chapters 1 and 2 for optimal brain function:

- Try to eat good protein sources throughout the day, including for breakfast and especially if you tend to have a 4pm slump.
- Make sure you have a varied diet that includes a range of B vitamins and other energy-producing nutrients.
- If you are regularly low in focus, concentration and energy, and particularly if you are stressed or vegan, take a good-quality multivitamin and mineral supplement with high levels of B vitamins.
- Add lecithin granules to food such as the Omega-rich Bircher Muesli on page 120, or yoghurt, cereals or soups.
- Observe your breathing habits to focus on the releasing exhalation.
- Take regular breaks.
- See Chapter 7 for good sleep quality.

Part Four

RECIPES FOR A STABLE AND HAPPY MOOD

CHAPTER 4

MOOD MAINTENANCE

We all feel blue from time to time, but when sadness or low motivation are regular visitors, looking at the factors we need to create and sustain good mood are vital. Much of our mood relies on our ability to be kind to ourselves. This self-compassion may come less easily to those who look after others or are not in the habit of recognizing that they deserve kindness and compassion.

Acknowledging this through time taken to nourish yourself with good food is an important first step. Times of low mood and even depression can signal the need for all the support recommended in the previous chapters, but we can also add in some very specific nutrients and foods that can help to regulate mood, keep the highs and lows at bay and feel on top of your emotional wellbeing.

On the list below, tick the symptoms that are familiar and persistent for you:

- Low mood.
- Lack of motivation for and pleasure in your usual activities and interests.
- Poor concentration.
- Difficulty making decisions.
- Disturbed appetite – either loss of or increased.

- Disturbed sleep – either sleeplessness or oversleeping, or often feeling unrefreshed by sleep.
- Tiredness.
- Decreased sexual energy (libido).
- Feelings of worthlessness and hopelessness.
- Anxiety.
- Physical symptoms that do not respond to treatment, such as headaches, digestive disorders and chronic pain.

If you ticked five or more of the above symptoms you may be suffering from a degree of depression, but the label is not our focus here, this chapter is about maintaining a balance and supporting a good mood.

Why do I feel this way?

Your body's ability to maintain mood and motivation depends on blood sugar balance, coping with stress and the nutrient building blocks for neurotransmitters, as we have explored in previous chapters.

Achieving a positive and buoyant mood (as well as other brain functions like cognition, focus and memory) also depends significantly on the health of your nerve cells. The efficiency at which messages travel along your nerves and through your brain is largely dictated by the condition of your brain cells, or neurons, and their casing. Each neuron has a protective sheath around it called myelin, which is broken up at intervals. Messages literally bounce from one of these intervals to the next, and when the message reaches the end of the neuron, it needs to be relayed across the tiny gap between the cells known as the synapse. To make this possible, chemicals called neurotransmitters (for example serotonin and dopamine, which we looked at in the last chapter) are released from the first cell. These cross the gap and dock into the next cell, transporting the message across. In order to retain optimum brain function, you need to provide your body with the raw materials – a constant supply of proteins, enzymes, salts and other molecules such as glucose and calcium ions – that it needs to produce healthy neurons and neurotransmitters.

In this chapter we are going to add in the all-important essential fatty acids (EFAs) – mainly focusing on omega 3 fatty acids (with some omega 6) – that play an important role in the health of brain cells. Picking up and utilizing our mood-enhancing neurotransmitters relies to a great extent on the various types of fat and their ratios in each fatty nerve cell membrane.

As we've discussed, but more importantly probably know from experience, when we feel even a little low, we are more likely to reach for a bar of chocolate than a bunch of carrots. It is well-researched that when we are stressed we crave sugar and fats for instant fuel and because they soothe stressy appetite signals on alert in the brain. Sugar has been shown to raise dopamine to give us a reward of feeling 'happy' as a quick fix that enables us to keep going, but unlike sugars, although fats can soothe agitated brain chemistry, they do not set up a cycle of craving and addiction. The sugar and fat combination we can crave is commonly found in the form of cakes, biscuits, pastries and crisps – yes, crisps and chips are savoury but, along with the other examples, it is the starchy carbohydrates in the potatoes (and also in the flour of the other foods mentioned) that we crave.

Many people assume that all fat is bad for them, but in fact our brains are made up largely of fats that they use for communication, so eating too little fat can have a noticeable impact on your moods. The key to good mood maintenance and body health is identifying which fats are your friends and which you should only eat in small doses.

Fats – good and bad...

The type of fats that we eat have a considerable impact on our health. There are three main types of dietary fat (also known as lipids): triglycerides, phospholipids and sterols (such as cholesterol).

Most body fats and almost all the fats we eat are triglycerides, the most common type of fat. Triglycerides can be either saturated or unsaturated, which refers to their chemical structure.

Saturated fats – those mainly found in animal products such as meat, butter and dairy foods, as well as coconut – are more rigid in structure than unsaturated fats and can be identified as those that remain solid at room temperature. Although these have been deemed 'unhealthy', there is still no conclusive evidence that they contribute to heart disease or other diseases, unless eaten with sugar or in processed meats (where the nitrate preservatives are the damaging aspects) or when omega 3 levels (see below) are too low in your diet. We need some saturated fats in our diets for cell communications, steroid hormones and vitamin D production, which are all important aspects of mood; we just don't need them in massive amounts.

Considered to be far more healthy than saturated fats, unsaturated fats are liquid at room temperature and can be further sub-divided into monounsaturated and polyunsaturated fats. Polyunsaturated fats is another name for essential fatty acids (EFAs), which we already know perform important structural and functional jobs in the body (see below). Monounsaturated fats are found in foods such as olive oil, avocados, nuts, peanuts and sesame seeds and are part of the traditional Mediterranean Diet, contributing to its well-researched properties of being anti-inflammatory, heart-protective and brain-supportive. They are semi-solid at room temperature, for example, they are seen as the sediment in olive oil on a cold day.

Let your skin be your judge

Your skin can provide a good indication of whether you are giving your whole body enough EFAs. Your body sees skin as less important than your other organs, and so it is last in line for receiving nutrients. Although dry skin can be a symptom of numerous underlying conditions, it won't hurt to increase your EFAs when it is showing signs of dehydration. That way, you can also be sure that your other organs, including your brain, are getting ample EFAs.

On the list below, tick any of the symptoms that you experience regularly:

- dry skin
- acne
- dermatitis
- eczema
- psoriasis
- allergies
- fatigue
- cracked nails
- dry, limp hair
- aching joints/arthritis
- depression
- high blood pressure.

If you suffer from any of the above symptoms, your diet could be lacking in EFAs and you may need to consider taking a supplement to boost your levels.

EFA families – omega 3 and 6

EFAs are converted in the body (with the help of certain vitamins and minerals) into more concentrated versions of the fats and other substances. These are then put to very good use in balancing hormones, keeping skin soft and much more. However, it is the role of the EFAs in ensuring that brain cells and neurotransmitters work efficiently that makes them such an important factor in maintaining stable moods and optimal brain power.

There are two families of EFAs: omega 3 and omega 6 (see below). In today's typical diet, it is common to have a higher intake of omega 6 fats than omega 3, yet for optimum health and stable moods, you need a balance of the two to keep communication going across cell membranes.

Essential fats are also needed to help break the vicious cycle of an exaggerated stress response. The fats found in foods such as oily fish, nuts and seeds help improve the health of every cell in your body; by doing this, they ensure that the substances that go in and out of each cell (for example, water, nutrients, hormonal messages and waste products) are properly regulated. These fats also moderate the body's production of natural inflammatory substances, which in excess encourage the release of too much cortisol, which as we know is not good for maintaining good mood (see page 46).

Omega 3

Omega 3 EFAs are found in the form DHA (docosahexaenoic acid) and EPA (eicosapentaenoic acid) in oily fish such as mackerel, trout, herring, pilchards, sardines, salmon and anchovies. These are the forms that we use easily in the body for cell membrane production and reducing inflammation, and are particularly important for emotional and mental health.

It is no coincidence that in societies such as those in the Arctic Circle or islands such as Taiwan, where people live on traditional fish-based diets, there are significantly lower incidences of heart disease and depression than in most Western nations. Scientists have actually found that lower consumption of omega 3 fatty acids correlates with increasing rates of depression. Indeed, one report showed that rates of depression in North America and Europe are 10 times higher than those in Taiwan.

Plant foods have omega 3 fats, too – in pumpkin and hemp seeds, walnuts and flaxseed oil – but these are in the alpha-linoleic acid form that need converting many times before we can use them as DHA and EPA. This conversion may be compromised in those with chronic stress or with 'atopic' inflammatory conditions such as asthma, acne, eczema, migraines, hayfever and arthritis.

Omega 6

Omega 6 essential fatty acids are found in vegetable oils such as sunflower and rapeseed oils (both of which are often used in margarines), and also evening primrose oil and borage (starflower) oil.

Omega 6 oils are high in the modern diet (coming from cereals, seed oils and bread) and have been shown to raise levels of endocannabinoids in the brain. Endocannabinoids increase appetite and dampen memory, mood, pain perception and energy (yep, the same system affected by cannabis and, yes, these effects similarly bring on 'the munchies' and are linked to weight gain). Eight weeks supplementation with krill oil (rich in both omega 3 fats and also phospholipids, which nourish brain chemistry) have been shown to reverse these metabolic dysfunctions.

Of all EFA plant sources, only flax and walnuts contain more omega 3 than 6, but in a form that still needs converting and that may only be as little as 5 per cent effective. It's not that you need to avoid these healthy foods, as they have other great health properties (such as soluble fibre for digestion, hormone-balancing lignans and zinc and vitamin E for skin health and healing), but be mindful when you may need to increase omega 3 through natural ingredients or supplements.

Supplementing EFAs

To improve your brain function, try taking an omega 3 oil supplement; most people do not need to supplement with omega 6 (as evening primrose oil, borage or starflower oil), as modern diets are much higher in omega 6 and lower in omega 3, particularly if they are plant-based. Many believe that this imbalance that has occurred since our diets became higher in refined vegetable and seed oils, has contributed to mental health issues and inflammation, such as the skin conditions mentioned above, but also is a root cause of digestive issues, heart disease and others.

Take omega 3 in the form of fish oils, krill oil or algae (vegan source):

- Fish oils: 2,000–4,000mg a day (usually 2–4 capsules) normal range with average of 325–330mg EPA/220–240mg DHA per 1,000mg.
- Krill oil: much less DHA and EPA but phospholipid form delivers to cells more easily, see labels.
- Algae rather than plant sources (e.g. flax, hemp) for vegetarians, as DHA/EPA needs to be converted from alpha-linoleic acid and is believed to be only 5 per cent effective. There are many good vegan DHA supplements on the market now.
- Also available with vitamin D3 for more mood support, especially in the winter months, see the box on page 118–19 for more information.

Research shows that supplementing with omega 3 oils may help reduce negative blood sugar effects of stress, reduce the anxiety associated with psychological stress and with mood and concentration, particularly krill oil, which protects the brain from the effects of stress.

A word about olive oil

Olive oil is one of the healthiest fats we can eat, especially if it is extra virgin and cold-pressed. It contains 7 per cent omega 6 fats, which, in a cold-pressed olive oil, retain all their healthy properties. The oil is made up of 75 per cent monounsaturated fat, which means that when used for cooking it is less susceptible to being damaged by heat and turning into a harmful trans fat (see page 113). For this reason, it is a much better oil to use for cooking than any of the polyunsaturated ones, such as sunflower oil, but just to medium heats – if you see the oil smoking, it can mean it has become oxidized and been damaged, so throw it away and start again. Several scientific studies have shown the traditional Mediterranean diet, which is high in olive oil, protects against many illnesses, including heart disease, in part because it is believed that there is a potent anti-inflammatory component in olive oil, oleocanthal.

Trans fats and hydrogenated fats

EFAs are very sensitive to damage from a combustion process called oxidation, which can transform 'good' fats into what is known as a trans-fatty acid (an unhealthy fatty acid), so high-EFA oils such as seed and nut oils shouldn't be used for cooking. This change that can occur in any fat has dramatic effects on the way it can be used in the body and ultimately on our health, including our mood and memory. If the fats that have already been incorporated into body structures – for example, in cell membranes – are damaged by oxidation, the way those structures work is impaired.

To extend their shelf-life, many processed oils, margarines and convenience foods have been heated and treated, forming trans fats. A manmade form, hydrogenated fats, are a type of trans fat that have been processed to make polyunsaturates (liquid oils, such as sunflower oil) and becomes solid at room temperature – such as in margarine. This type of fat used to be touted as 'healthy' but is now known to be detrimental to health.

Hydrogenated fats have to be declared on labels as they are manmade, unlike trans fats that occur naturally. Eat unprocessed foods, cooked from scratch and steamed, poached, baked or grilled/broiled rather than fried or barbecued. If you do eat processed foods, check the labels to make sure they don't mention hydrogenated fat, and store cold-pressed oils and fresh seeds in the fridge, where they are protected from rancidity caused by heat, light and oxygen exposure.

A GUIDE TO INCLUDING MOOD-SUPPORTING FATS IN YOUR DIET

- Have 1 tablespoon of cold-pressed, unrefined seed oil daily on salads, stirred into soups, on porridge, in smoothies or just taken neat.
- Add pumpkin, sunflower, sesame, hemp and flaxseeds (see page 57) to cereals, soups, yoghurt, porridge and salads daily; raw is better than toasted as the omega fatty acids are polyunsaturated and easily damaged by heat. You can also grind these seeds to use as a powder.
- Use whole pumpkin, sunflower and sesame seeds (black sesame seeds are lovely) as snacks.
- Flax and chia seeds can be soaked overnight in enough water to cover them and added to smoothies or cereals, see page 114.
- Eat oil-rich fish (such as salmon, mackerel, sardines, trout, herring) at least three times a week. If you do not eat fish or are vegan or vegetarian, you may need to consider a supplement, see page 112. Tuna and swordfish are not on this

list as they contain the toxic metal mercury, which can disrupt signals in the nervous system.

- Avoid all refined, processed oils, including processed foods containing them (look out for hydrogenated fat in the list of ingredients) and trans fats, those created by frying, barbecuing and charring. It is best to avoid fried foods as much as possible and grill/broil, bake, poach or steam instead.
- Use olive oil for cooking at low–medium heats only and coconut oil or butter at higher heats as these saturated fats (solid at room temperature) are more stable in the presence of heat and light. The fats in olive oil are mainly monounsaturated (between saturated and polyunsaturated) and have a potent anti-inflammatory action that helps protect us from the effects of chronic stress.
- When eating saturated fats in meat or dairy, choose organic where possible and grass-fed, rather than grain-fed, as well as free-range for the most healthy fat profile; these animals will have higher omega 3 intake, and therefore their meat will have a higher omega 3 content.

How inflammation impacts mood

EFAs and antioxidants are important features in our diet (and supplements when we need them) in large part because of their anti-inflammatory action. Mood and mental health issues have been more recently acknowledged as often having inflammation as part of their picture, and when we consider that inflammation is an important protective part of the stress response, this makes sense. It's there when we're on that 'alert to danger' mode, as our bodies expect the big physical reaction of fight or flight, so inflammatory pathways are turned on to protect us from the injury that could well happen. The trouble is they can stay turned on, particularly if low-level stress continues, and therefore so does low-grade inflammation, which is both exhausting and has been shown to bring down mood and motivation to conserve energy. We'll look at this more in relation to the gut in the next chapter.

Antioxidants

One of the most important ways by which we can reduce inflammation and protect the brain is through a good level of antioxidant nutrients eaten daily. It is important to ensure that your nerves are well protected. The rich fat content in the neuron's protective myelin sheath and in cell membranes makes them particularly susceptible to attack by oxidants. These byproducts of burning oxygen for fuel are like 'sparks' and are produced by anything burning – including cigarettes, cooking fat and petrol, and even by our own body's process of burning food to produce energy inside our body cells. Oxidant sparks damage cells, thereby making the body more vulnerable to disease and accelerating the ageing process, which includes a decline in nerve health. The body therefore needs a good supply of antioxidant nutrients (from a base of plenty of fresh vegetables and fruit in your diet) which protect it by quenching or neutralizing these damaging oxidising factors, hence 'anti'-oxidant. The brain creates a huge amount of energy, so it pumps out a lot of 'exhaust fumes' or oxidizing, unstable molecules that can damage brain cells. Antioxidants are a natural part of our diet to address this; researchers have found that people with higher levels of antioxidants in their blood tend to score better on memory tests.

Key antioxidants are vitamin E (contained in seeds, nuts, spinach, sweet potato and avocado), vitamin C (fruits and vegetables), vitamin A and beta-carotene (orange or red foods), glutathione (onions and garlic) and anthocyanidins (berries and beetroot/beet) found in many foods and drinks throughout the natural world, such as garlic, green tea, red wine, ginger, turmeric and thyme oil. See the list of antioxidant-rich foods on page 144 for more examples.

Anti-inflammatory/antioxidant supplements

So when stress is high (and particularly if you have any of the inflammatory conditions mentioned on page 109) you might want to take an antioxidant/anti-inflammatory nutrient complex, especially if you burn greater amounts of energy by exercising a lot. Look for any of the antioxidant substances in the following table; there are many different varieties, so ask a nutritional therapist for advice if you need to, as they all have different actions. Those marked with an asterisk* are known to support good blood sugar balance, too.

Ingredients of a good anti-inflammatory/antioxidant supplement		
Vitamins A, E, C*	Minerals zinc* and selenium	Carotenoids: beta carotene, alpha carotene, lycopene, astaxanthin, lutein
Cinnamon*	Resveratrol	Co-enzyme Q10*
Bromelain	Quercetin	Alpha lipoic acid*
Turmeric/active agent curcumin*	Green tea extract/ catechins*	Berry extracts/ anthocyanins*
Citrus bioflavonoids	Hespiridin	Rutin
Carotenoids; beta carotene, lutein, astaxanthin, lycopene	Green 'superfoods', e.g. chlorella, spirulina, chlorophyll	Herbs like Boswellia, Goldenseal, Olive Leaf and Cat's Claw

VITAMIN D – BRINGING THE SUNSHINE TO SAD SUFFERERS

One key mood nutrient that is bound up with the fats in our bodies is vitamin D. Often called the 'sunshine nutrient', we produce this fat-soluble antioxidant in our bodies, signalled by sunlight on our skin; cortisol (stress) affects our ability to take vitamin D into our cells to use. It is crucial for mental health and also for bone mineralization and immunity. Low levels of vitamin D from lower light levels in the winter contributes to Seasonal Affective Disorder (SAD), which is also related to low serotonin levels – lower light levels means lower levels of natural production of the hormone melatonin (needed for sleep) and so we use up serotonin to create melatonin. Most SAD sufferers experience extreme tiredness and sleep more than usual, as they become less motivated because of their lowered serotonin. They also tend to have a significant increase in appetite and therefore weight during the winter months.

Making sure you get outside and get active in winter is crucial for quality of life in many ways. The darker your skin tone, the more sun exposure on your skin you will need to produce the same amount of vitamin D as a fairer-skinned person, as pigments are there to protect you from sunlight radiation damage in hotter countries. Cloud cover in the Northern Hemisphere tends to mean little UV light gets through anyway, so a vitamin D supplement is advised for most people in the winter months, especially if you work indoors or cover up. However, good natural sources of vitamin D include:

- Direct sunlight is the best source; at least 15 minutes a day without sunscreen but before any reddening occurs.
- We can obtain some vitamin D from food, with high

amounts found in mackerel, salmon, trout, herring and moderate amounts in eggs. Cow's milk and other dairy foods are fortified with vitamin D in the US but not the UK.

- The vegetarian form, vitamin D2, works less effectively than the D3 form, with spray versions being best absorbed in tissues within the mouth.
- A supplementation range of 2,000-10,000IUs a day is safe; 2,000 is common in high-strength supplements.

A ray of hope

The control centres in our brains that determine our moods and daily rhythms are governed in part by the amount of light that enters our eyes. During the night, or in darkness, melatonin production increases, making us sleepy. When day breaks and our eyes are exposed to natural light, melatonin production stops. During the dark winter days, therefore, the control mechanism for melatonin release changes. It appears that SAD sufferers are especially sensitive to this change. Light therapy, or phototherapy, is a treatment for SAD that involves daily exposure to high-intensity, broad-spectrum artificial light from a light box, which suppresses the production of melatonin and raises that of serotonin.

Building on the recipes and advice from the previous three chapters, now we are going to focus on how to include plenty of healthy fats and antioxidants in your daily diet to ensure a balanced, happy mood.

Omega-rich
Bircher Muesli

This home-made muesli takes seconds to prepare, all to your own specifications, and you can then store a batch ready for breakfast at home, for your commute, to eat at your desk or as a great afternoon snack. This is the Bircher version of muesli, where the ingredients are soaked overnight to break down the fibres in the grains that are difficult for us to digest. Soaking the nuts and seeds also helps you digest and receive their rich EFAs.

Cinnamon and coconut are both included in this recipe for their high antioxidant status. The MCT fats in coconut are medium-chain triglycerides, plant forms of saturated fats that we cannot store in the body as fat, but are potent antioxidants and similar to the saturated fats in breast milk. They also support blood sugar balance (see page 39).

200 g (7 oz) oat flakes
200 g (7 oz) barley flakes
200 g (7 oz) rye flakes
4 dessertspoons unsweetened
   dessicated/dried coconut
2 dessertspoons sunflower seeds
2 dessertspoons pumpkin seeds

3 dessertspoons dried fruit
   (prunes or figs are best) or
   fresh berries
1 teaspoon ground cinnamon
good-quality apple juice or plain
   yoghurt, to serve

1   Mix all the dry ingredients together in a large storage container with a lid. You can add any other nuts, seeds or dried fruits you like; fresh berries are best added just before serving. Good healthfood stores also sell a range of other grains (some are best puffed, such as quinoa, as they are inedible raw) that you can add to the mixture. Store in a cool place.

2   To prepare, soak a bowlful, or any container you want to transport it in, with good-quality apple juice or yoghurt to cover, overnight. You can also eat as a dry muesli with any milk or yoghurt, if you prefer.

Seatown Kedgeree

This version of kedgeree is a variation on the Versatile Rice Salad on page 92, but with more emphasis on the oily fish and seeds for their omega 3 fats. Watercress is included here because it is a strong provider of antioxidants, particularly the fat-soluble carotenoids that protect our fatty brains and the blood-brain barrier at the base of the skull – the point between the brain and the rest of the body that needs constant nourishment. Watercress and parsley are also great sources of vitamin C, which protects this barrier and other fluids around the brain, too.

This dish can be made with eggs as well as, or instead of, the fish – as a classic Indian kedgeree that would have been served up for breakfast in Victorian times. Some people like peas, some do not, but green peas are higher in protein than many other beans – almost as high as soy beans, which here can be a protein alternative to the fish and eggs for vegans and vegetarians, but bear in mind that they lack the omega 3 fats you will find in those.

If you are including eggs, you can buy those called 'omega 3 eggs', where the chicken feed will have been enriched with omega 3 fats, but bear in mind that these are not always free-range or organic. It is better to buy eggs from chickens who have been allowed to roam freely (check out your local farms), for their welfare but also because they will have had a diet and exercise that tends to naturally increase omega 3 fats in their eggs.

Serves 2

100 g (3½ oz) brown rice (basmati if possible), or a combination of brown and wild rice

1 onion, finely diced

splash of olive oil and knob of butter, for frying

2 cooked smoked mackerel, trout or salmon fillets

handful of seeds – sunflower, pumpkin or sesame, or a combination

handful of watercress, roughly chopped

handful of cooked green peas (optional)

1 dessertspoon finely chopped parsley

½ teaspoon curry powder

1   Cook the rice following the packet instructions.

2   Gently cook the onion in the olive oil and butter – be careful not to let it brown too much.

3   Remove any skin from the fish and break it up. When the rice is cooked, fold all the ingredients in together and serve with a fresh spinach salad.

Smoked Fish Pâté

This is an amazingly quick, easy dish to make for lunch, breakfast, as a snack or even a starter for a dinner party.

You may be surprised to see the inclusion of butter here as well as the omega 3 fats in the mackerel; this illustrates how having some saturated fat with plenty of omega 3 oils in our diets is not an unhealthy choice. In fact, butter provides the fat-soluble antioxidant vitamins A and D, as well as butyric acid that feeds gut cells. Also here we have specified full-fat (not skimmed or 0% fat) yoghurt to benefit from the brain-satisfying presence of the fats in the natural ratio that our body expects to receive dairy and at which the liver can process. Try to use organic to avoid ingesting hormones and medications from commerically reared livestock.

Serves 2

150 g (5 oz) smoked mackerel fillets, skin removed

2 spring onions/scallions, chopped

50 g (2 oz) butter

50 g (2 oz) plain, full-fat Greek yoghurt

1 dessertspoon freshly squeezed lemon juice

1 tablespoon chopped parsley

1   Blend all the ingredients together in a blender to create either a slightly rougher or smoother texture, depending on your taste. Place in a bowl and chill in the fridge until you are ready to serve.

2   Eat with rye or rice crackers, or crudités. If serving to friends or family, you could garnish this with slices of lemon and sprigs of parsley.

Trout with Sunflower Seeds

This is a wonderful variation on a classic dinner-party dish – trout with almonds – so any nut or seed can be used. You can use any oily fish you like instead of trout, but do make sure that it is fresh. This is a beautifully simple way to create a protein- and omega-3-rich basis for a meal, to which you can add any salad or vegetable side dish for plenty of antioxidants.

Serves 4

4 whole trout, filleted

2 lemons

1 tablespoon olive oil

3 tablespoons sunflower seeds

1   Preheat the oven to 200°C/400°F/Gas Mark 6.

2   Lay the fish in an ovenproof baking dish. Cut the lemons in half and squeeze the juice over the fish. Drizzle over the olive oil. Place in the oven and bake for 20 minutes, turning them over once halfway through cooking.

3   Toss the sunflower seeds in a dry frying pan until they are lightly toasted. Just before serving the fish, sprinkle the seeds over the top of each trout.

Thai-style Noodle Soup

There are so many variations on the theme of Asian-style soups that you can experiment with: hotter, vegetarian, with or without noodles. This recipe is for a filling meal in itself – you can substitute the prawns with slices of fish, chicken breast, beef or tofu. If you decide to make extra for freezing, don't add the noodles into the frozen batch; instead, cook them at the last minute when you're serving it.

This is a rich, dense, antioxidant-packed dish, with the buckwheat noodles providing a great grain-free alternative to wheat noodles, because buckwheat is actually a seed rather than a grain. You could use rice noodles instead, but they are purely starch and miss out on the protein, antioxidants, minerals, vitamins and soluble fibre that buckwheat contains. They have very little fat, though, made up for here by the coconut milk, added for deep satisfaction and the immune-supporting antioxidant fat, lauric acid.

Serves 4

150 g (5 oz) udon buckwheat noodles

extra virgin olive oil, for cooking

2 teaspoons Thai green curry paste

2 cloves garlic, finely chopped

1 lemongrass stalk, sliced into 6

2½ cm (1 inch) piece of fresh root ginger, sliced

250 g (9 oz) fresh prawns or tofu

8 baby corn, sliced

8 spring onions/scallions, sliced

2 carrots, peeled and sliced

12 mangetout/snow peas

1 x 400 ml (14 fl oz) can coconut milk

3–4 kaffir lime leaves

a few sprigs of fresh coriander/cilantro

1   Cook the noodles following the packet instructions, rinse well
    with cold water and divide between four large bowls.

2   In a large pan, heat the olive oil and stir in the curry paste, garlic,
    lemongrass and ginger. Add a tablespoon of water. Toss in the
    prawns or tofu and stir for a few minutes until they are pink and
    cooked through. Fish them out with a slotted spoon and lay
    them on the noodles.

3   Add the rest of the vegetables, including the mangetout, to the
    pan, stirring them in the spices for a couple of minutes. Pour
    in the coconut milk and add the lime leaves. Add a couple of
    canfuls of water, bring to the boil and leave to simmer for 12–15
    minutes, or until the vegetables are cooked. At the last minute,
    stir in half the chopped coriander. Ladle the soup evenly over
    the noodles and cooked prawns/tofu and garnish with the rest
    of the coriander.

Chicken or Tofu Sesame Stir-fry

This chicken/tofu and vegetable stir-fry is fabulous served with rice or noodles and sprinkled with sesame seeds – the black ones look great and their dark colour shows their higher levels of the sesamoid antioxidants. Sesame seeds also contain high levels of vitamin E.

For meat-eaters, choosing free-range and organic chicken here ensures a better fat profile as it will have received the movement and diet to increase its omega 3 content. It is both nutritionally and ethically intelligent to pay more for meat that is healthier for both you and the animal – pay more and buy less, relying on more vegetarian sources of protein and fat.

Serves 4

2 chicken breasts, lean and skinless, or about 180 g (6 oz) firm tofu

1 tablespoon soy sauce

2½ cm (1 inch) fresh root ginger, finely sliced

1 clove garlic, finely sliced

2 dessertspoons olive oil

1 teaspoon Chinese five spice

handful of sugarsnap peas or mangetout/snow peas

1 onion, chopped

1 red pepper, deseeded and cut into strips

1 carrot, cut into thin strips

1 tablespoon finely chopped coriander/cilantro

2 tablespoons black sesame seeds

1   Slice the chicken (or tofu) into thin strips, place in a bowl along with the soy sauce, sliced ginger and garlic and mix well to coat. If you have time, leave to marinate for 2–3 hours.

2   Heat a wok or frying pan and add one dessertspoon of the olive oil. Quickly stir in the marinated chicken/tofu along with the marinade, tossing continuously until cooked through. Remove the chicken/tofu with a slotted spoon (leaving any liquid in the pan), and set aside.

3   Add the other dessertspoon of olive oil to the pan to heat. Put the Chinese five spice, all the prepared vegetables and the coriander into the pan. Toss quickly and add 2 tablespoons of water to steam fry. Stir well on a high heat for about 2 minutes. Then return the chicken/tofu to the pan and reheat until you are sure it is hot all the way through, without letting the vegetables become soft. Scatter with sesame seeds and serve.

Dahl

Dahl simply means 'lentils', so this is just one of probably dozens of recipes using this Indian staple. Lentils are a good source of starchy carbohydrates, with 29 per cent protein, so they make a complete meal or a great side dish. This version is very quick and easy to prepare and freezes well, ensuring a ready supply of the antioxidants in the garlic, olive oil, onion and spices. As well as the quicker instructions here, you can also simply place all of the ingredients in a slow cooker/crockpot and let them cook for 8 hours on a low heat; this keeps the antioxidants intact.

Serves 3

1 mug of orange split lentils
1 onion, chopped
5 cloves garlic, crushed
1 teaspoon olive oil
1 teaspoon ground coriander
1 teaspoon ground cumin

1 teaspoon turmeric
chilli powder, to taste (optional)
3 mugs of water
400 g (14 oz) can chopped
   tomatoes

1   Wash the lentils thoroughly in a sieve/fine-mesh strainer and remove any little stones. In a large saucepan, soften the onion and garlic in the olive oil and spices. Do not allow the mixture to brown – if necessary, add a little water. You can add chilli powder to taste if you would like the dahl to be hot as well as spicy. Add the lentils, water and tomatoes and leave to simmer over a low heat for about 1 hour, stirring regularly to make sure the lentils do not stick on the bottom. If the dahl starts to become too thick, add a little more water.

2   Serve with brown basmati rice and steamed broccoli.

Which lifestyle changes help maintain good mood?

Nourishing yourself with good food is an important first step in helping to stabilize your mood, but just as important is taking time out from constantly doing things to attend to all of your physical and mental needs, too.

Kind attention

Much of our mood is determined by the habits of our minds and it is pretty common for the modern mind to be overwhelmed by information. If you are under chronic stress, dominated by fears and prone to worry, your mind will be stuck in this hypervigilant 'constant alert' state that doesn't allow it to rest and find peace, which is a condition often related to depressive states. This constant agitation uses up swathes of brain-energy and leaves you with the demotivated state that is such a deep part of depression.

Mindfulness is the dedicated practice of experiencing the present moment, simply as it is, without self-criticism or judgement. Whether practised as a formal meditation or within daily life, it helps us to step away from constant ruminations, such as going through scenarios in our minds or having feelings dominated by worry. There are many mindfulness courses and apps available now to help you retrain your mind from busy to quiet.

Active relaxation

Fully letting go and relaxing is the recovery phase that all aspects of our mind-body need on a daily basis, not just on holiday once every six months. Relaxation that fully allows the mind to be soothed and come to a feeling of safety, and therefore peace, is conscious and involves an awareness of the whole of our body and being – where we are, in the here and now. We do not get this from slumping in front of the TV, which actually keeps a vigilant brain on a high alert, with the quick movements, noises and constantly changing light and colour stimuli.

Activities where we 'don't do' and so 'undo' are an important part of mental health. These can be walking in nature, mindful movement within yoga, t'ai chi or qigong, meditation, creative pursuits such as drawing, colouring, sewing or knitting, or even simply taking a bath and being present to the sensations. For extra benefit, try adding Epsom salts to a bath – they are well-known for their deep soothing of the nervous system, support of tissue healing and for reducing muscle soreness and pain, including after exercise. Just add a cup or two (or more!) of Epsom salts to a warm bath and soak for at least 20 minutes. The salts are magnesium sulphate so you are both absorbing calming magnesium (see page 54–5) and detoxifying sulphur (see page 158).

TOP TIPS FOR MAINTAINING YOUR MOOD

On top of the blood-sugar-balancing, stress-reducing and nutrient-providing advice in the first three chapters, to give your mood an extra boost, try:

- At least three times a week, eat pumpkin, sunflower, sesame, hemp and flaxseeds and/or oil-rich fish such as salmon, mackerel, sardines, tuna or herring.
- Take an omega 3 oil supplement.
- Ensure your diet is chock-full of antioxidant vegetables, fruit, garlic, ginger, spices and other foods from nature.
- Consider taking an antioxidant supplement if you have an inflammatory condition, high stress and/or you exercise to a high level.

Part Five

RECIPES TO SOOTHE THE GUT

CHAPTER 5

SOOTHING BELLY STRESS

Phrases like 'I feel it in my gut' and 'I have butterflies in my tummy' show just how much our emotions and mental states show up in our bellies. Not simply another aspect of mood health, the condition of and voices from our gut are a fundamental part of how our brains and bodies regulate and respond to how we feel about the world around us. We don't need to be suffering digestive complaints to need to take care of our gastrointestinal (GI) tract, or gut.

Although your brain may seem a long way from your gut, liver and bowels, it does in fact rely on them in order to function effectively. How you feel is, to a large extent, dictated by how well your body is digesting food, absorbing nutrients, detoxifying and eliminating waste, but also the amazing continual communication bi-way that we are only just beginning to understand – the gut-brain axis.

Reducing sugar, increasing fibre and antioxidants through eating more vegetables and reducing inflammation in the gut via EFAs and antioxidants is a great foundation for gut health, and in this chapter we will explore how and which other measures can support your mood via your belly.

To gauge your digestive health before we get started, tick on the list below any symptoms that you experience regularly:

- Difficulty self-soothing.
- Bad breath.
- Frequent burning sensation when you urinate.
- Fullness in stomach.
- Difficulty digesting fatty foods.
- Flatulence or bloating or excessive belching.
- Diarrhoea.
- Fewer than one bowel movement a day.
- Recurrent headaches.
- Sensitivity to chemicals, pollution, cigarette smoke, perfumes.
- Spots or acne.
- Poor tolerance of alcohol.

If you suffer from any of the above, you may well not be digesting or detoxifying properly, but also, maybe surprisingly, the first symptom here refers to how important gut health is to our ability to find calm and mental adaptability.

Why do I feel this way?

How well we break down and absorb food not only determines the nutrients we receive, but also the health of our whole digestive tract. The workings of your liver – your body's main organ of detoxification – are inextricably bound with this tube that runs from mouth to anus, otherwise known as your digestive tract. The health of your gut – its bacterial environment or 'microbiome'– has considerable consequences for the rest of your body. So your gut and your liver together have an impact on your overall health, including your mood and energy. Your mood, energy and stress levels also play a significant role in the efficacy of your gut and liver function.

The gut as 'Second Brain'

Much of the mood connection with the gut is through the branch of the nervous system housed through your entire digestive tract. This enteric nervous system ('enteric', meaning of the gut) or ENS is often referred to as our 'Second Brain' as it can act independently from our central nervous system (brain and spinal cord) and has as many brain cells (neurons) as a cat's brain! It can feel, respond and remember, and it can play a large part in our decision-making and behaviour, although it isn't actually capable of conscious thought!

Much of the work of the ENS is the daily grind of digestion, but it also senses our intuitive and instinctive feelings of how we feel about a person or situation – hence the 'I have a feeling in my gut'. This information is constantly feeding back up to the brain via the vagus nerve and tells us how to respond moment to moment. Most of our decision-making is about whether we like or dislike something or someone, and depending on our conclusion we move closer (approach or allow) or back off (withdraw or protect). Much of this will be unconscious, unless we choose to really pay attention to our gut and bring our relationship with our gut feelings and reactions to consciousness.

Much research shows that this 'trusting your gut' is an important part of our survival responses, as it helps us to learn what we deem to be safe or unsafe and react immediately. Problems can arise when we are playing out habits and patterns that we learned in our most formative, younger years – up to the age of seven. This is when we are laying down how we see the world without consciously processing it, as 'somatic markers' – felt as emotional responses in the gut. If this feels unsafe, we can end up playing out vigilant and self-defensive strategies because they are the only ones we have; whether they are relevant or not any more.

The Gut-Brain Axis

This is where the gut feeds into our stress responses. If we are programmed or wired for constant self-protection, the hypervigilance described on page 43 can be a way of life. This constant fear-based look-out happens from the primal, reptilian part of our brains, and when we consider that in the two-way communication line of the gut-to-brain, 80 per cent of information is moving bottom up – from our gut feelings to our brain responses – we can see why we can go into automatic patterns of anxiety, overwhelm and freeze.

This pathway is known as the Gut-Brain Axis (GBA) and is an important part of mood regulation. Understanding how soothing the gut wall and supporting the gut environment affects our mental health is something that is just beginning to be fully understood, but we know that the gut produces the same neurotransmitters that we have in the brain, just in larger amounts. It is reckoned that about 90 per cent of the body's serotonin and 50 per cent of its dopamine works within the gut and is part of the signalling through the GBA. These chemicals also play roles in digestion, determining which parts move and stop to allow the passage of food, which is why one of the side-effects of medications that alter brain chemistry can often be digestive upset.

The microbiome – your friendly bug colony

It is important to note that neurotransmitters in the gut and brain don't travel between these sites, but those in your digestive tract can still affect your mood. Scientists are just beginning to uncover the secrets behind this amazing signalling route – the gut microbiome or the colony of helpful bacteria that live in the mucosal lining of your gut.

In your gut there is 1.3–1.8kg (3–4lb) of live bacteria – more cells than in of your whole skin! In a healthy digestive tract these bacteria consist of about 80 per cent 'friendly' bacteria and 20 per cent 'bad' bacteria. The friendly 'probiotic' bacteria help keep the 'bad' and other invaders like yeasts (such as candida albicans) in check. Low probiotic bacteria have been associated with anxiety and depression, and stress has been shown to deplete their levels. This means a vicious cycle of stress that leaves us more prone to low mood and poor coping mechanisms. It is also known that the personal level of inflammation that stress can cause (see page 115) partly occurs via the gut – the less healthy a gut microbiome, the more likely you are to have inflammation throughout other parts of the body.

Research has shown that consuming probiotic foods and/or supplements might influence mood by reducing inflammatory immune components called cytokines that are running around the body, and the oxidative stress that they create, such as damage to tissues and also increasing our vulnerability to anxiety and depression. They can also increase tryptophan levels for serotonin production, normalize brain levels of stress hormones and possibly even regulate blood sugar levels. Recently, much research has demonstrated significant improvements in people suffering from depression, anger and anxiety, as well as lower levels of the stress hormone cortisol among healthy adults who are taking a daily probiotic supplement.

Probiotic levels are lowered by a diet that is high in sugar and refined foods, antibiotic and steroid medications, and stress. Many of the yeasts, parasites or harmful bacteria that can proliferate in an unhealthy gut may cause low-lying digestive symptoms such as bloating (if not more serious problems), and they can also subtly release toxins that affect mood. When a person in such a situation works with a professional health practitioner to eliminate the unwanted organisms and re-establish the levels of friendly bacteria, the improvement in mood and other symptoms can be remarkable.

Your body as a food processor

As we have seen, the healthier your gut environment, the more you can regulate mood and cope with life's ups and downs. Full digestion of food – its breakdown, absorption and assimilation into the body via the gut wall, and ultimately elimination of that we don't need (yes, healthy bowel movements!) – both relies on and affects the delicate optimal bacterial and pH (acid-alkaline) balance within your gut.

After the all-important first job of chewing your food to mix it with saliva, which starts to break down the food and kills off a few 'baddies', the food reaches your stomach, where a substance called hydrochloric acid continues the digestive process. The partially digested food then passes into the small intestine, where digestive enzymes and bile from the liver break it down further into small-enough particles to be absorbed across the intestinal lining. The remaining 'food' then passes into the large intestine, or colon, where some more absorption of nutrients takes place and what is left is prepared for elimination from the body. The nutrients that are absorbed are carried directly to the liver, where they are sorted out, pulled apart, repackaged and sent off for distribution around the body or back to the gut for elimination.

When digestion is working well, we hardly notice it, but when we experience variables of our diet, eating habits and body processes – what we eat, how much we eat, how well we are producing stomach acid and intestinal juices, how efficiently our gut is moving food along, the acidity of the gut, the balance of bacteria in the intestines, the amount of water present to support the process – there is plenty that can get knocked off course, for instance if we are stressed, eating too quickly, eating foods that upset our digestion or if we are dehydrated. If your diet consists of foods that are highly refined, high in animal or processed fats, low in fibre, laden with sugar or generally not as rich in nutrients as they could be, and you are also drinking too much coffee, tea or alcohol and not enough water between meals, you are stacking up the odds against good digestion and detoxification.

Stress doesn't just change the quality of your microbiome, it also halts the digestive processes immediately. As stress is survival mode, your body diverts most of its energy to dealing with the 'threat', rather than doing jobs that it perceives to be more long-term and so unimportant at that moment – one of which is digestion. So when you are stressed, none of the processes in the digestive tract are likely to be working efficiently, yet you are likely to still be eating food, which ends up not being processed properly. This can result in putrefied food hanging around and gases being produced that are a recipe for indigestion, bloating, constipation, diarrhoea, inflammatory bowel diseases and other digestive problems.

Detoxing

You only have to remember how low you felt on a Sunday, having consumed a large amount of alcohol the previous Friday night, to see what a dampening effect overloading your liver can have on your mood and energy. Or, if you are not much of a drinker, you may notice how overeating fatty, processed foods for a couple of days leaves you sluggish, lethargic and unmotivated.

In recent years, as 'detox' diets and programmes have become fashionable, it has been easy to forget that the body does not detoxify only when we 'go on a detox' – it does so every second we are alive. Supporting these processes is a key component of mood regulation.

It is not just how toxic a substance is that makes it harmful, but also how efficiently your body is able to process it. In a sensitive person, any number of substances – those that build up in the body and those that come from the outside – can act as toxins and interfere with the chemistry of the brain. The mechanisms that control the balance of neurotransmitters such as serotonin – how they are produced and then how efficiently they are transmitted – are so finely tuned that any slight interference caused by toxic overload is likely to disturb these processes.

If the liver is overloaded you also end up with an excess of oxidants in the body (see page 143) that damage cell membranes, which need to be healthy for the transmission of messages in the brain. Given that your mood is in part dictated by the transmission of messages using substances such as serotonin, an inefficient messaging system could well mean that your moods are not all they could be.

Toxic exposure

In addition to the nutrients carried to the liver from the digestive tract, any other substances that happen to get across the gut lining are also taken there. Unfortunately, these substances sometimes include toxins and food particles that have not been completely digested or that a less-than-healthy gut wall may have accidentally let through – especially if stress or other problems mean that you are not digesting food correctly. Our normal metabolic processes also produce chemicals within the body that need to be detoxified and eliminated.

We are all constantly exposed to countless external toxins. Our environments are increasingly filled with substances that

TOXINS

Toxins are internal and external substances that place a burden on the body's reserves. The work they represent for the liver depends not just on their inherent toxic properties but also on the body's ability to detoxify them.

What places a burden on the liver?

- Alcohol – a neurotoxin (it is harmful to the brain) that your liver will prioritize breaking down. If you drink, aim to have no more than four to six glasses of wine or shots of spirits per week and try to keep some weeks completely alcohol free.
- Prescription drugs – oral contraceptives, high-dose aspirin/acetaminophen, etc.
- Recreational drugs.
- Exposure to chemicals – pesticides, industrial chemicals, paints, solvents, fuels.
- A low-fibre, highly refined diet.
- Excessive fat, protein, calories.
- Bowel toxicity owing to poor detoxification and elimination.
- Dietary sources of oxidants – rancid oils, fried or charred foods.
- Stress – increases the amount of chemicals produced and broken down again by the liver for reactions: hormones, enzymes and neurotransmitters.

our bodies have to process in order to render them harmless. Toxins processed in the liver are passed through into the gut to be carried out of the body. If you are not eliminating waste via your bowels properly or regularly, the toxins are more likely to hang around and be circulated back around your body.

Nutrients for digestion and detoxification

By choosing foods and drinks that aid the digestive system rather than overload it, you can directly reduce the demands on your liver. The following are particularly important:

Fibre

One of the most important ways of supporting the liver is including plenty of fibre in your diet. Fibre is not just about having your morning prunes to stave off constipation (although they do work, see the Bircher muesli, page 120!). Having regular bowel movements is almost as important for your health as putting good food in your mouth, because it means that you are eliminating waste products effectively. Fibre not only keeps your gut moving, it also binds onto toxins in the gut and escorts them out of the body.

- Barley, beans (such as, borlotti, pinto, kidney, black-eyed, chickpeas, lentils), brown rice, buckwheat, fresh fruit, fresh vegetables, oats, rye, soaked seeds such as chia and flaxseeds; also pectin in carrots, apples and plums.

Antioxidants (see page 116)

This is a very important group of nutrients for supporting liver detoxification and healing the gut wall. Rich plant sources will also provide a variety of fibre sources, such as:

- Avocado, beetroot/beet, berries, broccoli, cabbage, carrots, garlic, grapes, green tea, kale, nuts, onions, peppers, prunes, seeds, sweet potatoes, tomatoes, watercress, herbs and spices.

Prebiotic foods

To promote 'friendly' bacteria, most fruit and vegetables provide the soluble fibre that feeds probiotic, beneficial bacteria, but certain foods have higher levels of this 'prebiotic' fibre, such as inulin.

- Asparagus, garlic, Jerusalem artichokes, onions, leeks, kiwi fruit, beans, bananas, psyllium husk powder (must be taken with plenty of water).

Fermented foods

Humans have a long historical relationship with fermented foods – fermentation was a process designed to preserve fresh ingredients long before we had fridges. Each culture has its own version of this method but each version helps support the gut environment by making it a hospitable place for good bacteria to flourish. Some (like yoghurt) also provide colonising bacteria directly. Many fermented foods are now available to buy in healthfood shops and good supermarkets.

- Live plain yoghurt, miso, sauerkraut, apple cider vinegar, kimchi, kefir, kombucha, sourdough, tamari.

Stomach acid support

If you aren't digesting food fully and have chronic stress, supporting your stomach acid levels can help. Although many with this profile have reflux or indigestion, this is often not caused by overacidity (where taking antacids can only worsen the issue), but low stomach acid, which means that undigested food in the stomach struggles to move into the small intestine and backs up into the throat, where there is no protective mucous lining (as in the stomach) and it causes a burning sensation. The natural acids in lemon juice and apple cider vinegar have long had traditional uses for digestive support, and when taken with meals directly or in dressings (see page 31) they both help to break down food and encourage bile flow, which is crucial for digestion of fats.

They also both support liver function, have strong natural antibiotic and antifungal action (to support the gut environment), are high in antioxidants and are potent anti-inflammatories. If you do find they burn, it is best to avoid them because you may have high stomach acid. You can neutralize this with bicarbonate of soda.

- Lemon juice, apple cider vinegar.

Soothing an irritated gut wall

The following foods and drinks are known to have calmative effects on the gut wall, so can help reduce feelings of pain, irritation, bloating and food intolerance (see more on this in the next chapter).

- Mint tea, camomile tea, fresh herbs, avocado; golden flaxseeds and chia seeds can be soaked overnight in enough water to cover them and then added to smoothies or cereals, or to the Omega-rich Bircher Muesli on page 120 – they produce a mucillage to coat and protect the gut wall.

Water for life

All cells contain and are surrounded by water – we need it for life and it is 'bound' in our bodies, so that we are made up of 55–60 per cent water but still have containment and structure. Digestive processes use up litres of water at a time, so to retain the fluidity of our cells and connective tissue, so vital to health and movement, we need to hydrate between meals. This tissue hydration also includes the fascia (type of connective tissue) around the viscera or digestive organs, which need to be able to move without stickiness or adhesion for full gut motility, which is how the muscles in the digestive tract move the food through it.

Many people with constipation find relief just by increasing their water intake. One of the large intestine's jobs is to draw water from the food that arrives there, in order to form faeces. If you do not drink enough water, your bowel will draw on as much as it can from the food, leaving a dry, compacted stool – that is, constipation. Alternatively, the large intestine can open gaps between cells in the gut wall to flood the gut with water taken from the bloodstream – diarrhoea.

Drinking lots of fluid at mealtimes can dilute stomach acid and digestive juices, so it is best to get your hydration at least an hour either side of meals. You can sip a little with meals without too much of an adverse effect, but most people who need to drink lots when they eat do so because they are not properly chewing and so not producing enough saliva to fully lubricate their food and be able to swallow it easily. Chewing more and drinking less is the best recipe for full digestion.

Although amounts such as 1.5–2 litres (2½–3½ pints) of water drunk throughout the day are recommended, the evidence for this is sketchy at best and is believed to have been propagated by bottled water companies. Yes, we do need to ensure hydration for all mind and body functions, but ideally this comes from a diet rich in water-filled vegetables and fruit, with the minerals present to ensure absorption. Drinking fluids between meals should probably be at a level of somewhere around 1.2 litres (2 pints), but this differs between people and circumstances; we need more if we are stressed, exercising a lot or the weather is hot.

It is best to drink charcoal filtered water – you can buy charcoal sticks online or more expensive filter systems. It is also great to get liquids from herbal or fruit teas, but sugary drinks – check the labels of so-called 'health waters' or fruit drinks – are known to create sugar dependence faster than by eating it. Juicing has become very popular, but this method can deliver a vast amount of sugar to the bloodstream quickly and may contribute to too-high bacterial levels in the small intestine. It is better to eat real food and hydrate. Remember that coffee and tea may dehydrate you depending on their strength.

Most herbal teas have calmative and healing properties for the digestive tract, but the following are particularly helpful:

- Chamomile tea – calms and soothes the ENS, as well as the central nervous system. It also acts as an anti-inflammatory on the gut wall, and has been shown to reduce conditions such as IBS and diarrhoea.
- Mint tea – peppermint has relaxant and antispasmodic properties and can help relieve cramps and spasms in the gastrointestinal tract, bile duct and gallbladder. It has been shown to help alleviate problems like bloating, stomach gas and flatulence.
- Spice-based teas – these are often cinnamon-based as the spice has been shown to lower temperatures in the stomach and help with digestive upset. Alongside ginger, which is anti-gas and nausea, it also regulates immune responses and blood sugar levels, which all help to keep the gut environment healthy and lower your sugar intake, which also helps gut health. These are common in Middle Eastern and Indian teas, where other digestive aids such as fennel, licorice, mint and cumin may also be included.
- Green tea and matcha – high catechin antioxidant levels heal the gut and support immune modulation from here. These are also great alternatives to lots of caffeine in coffee and black tea that may irritate the gut wall. They do contain some caffeine, but also soothing L-theanine (see page 56).

Supplements for gut health

The best way to 'recolonize' your gut with beneficial bacteria is to take a probiotic supplement that you can buy in a good healthfood shop. If you have deeper digestive or detoxification problems, this is best recommended by a nutritional therapist or naturopath, who can also arrange stool testing (via a laboratory) to ascertain exactly what you need.

Alternatively, eating plain yoghurt that is made with live cultures every day can give you a regular supply of probiotics. However, bear in mind that yoghurts or yoghurt drinks with added sugar usually cancel out any benefit, as sugar tends to feed the 'bad' bacteria.

We've discussed how probiotics have been shown to help reduce stress-related anxiety through signalling back up to the brain. Low levels are also linked to weight gain, depression and inflammation. Those with better levels of beneficial probiotic bacteria in their guts have been shown to be able to digest grains and beans more efficiently, with less gas and bloating.

Guide to buying probiotics

- Find a good-quality probiotic capsule or powder (see below) – add powders to yoghurt or smoothies or other cold foods that don't destroy the bacteria.
- Main strains are lactobacillus and bifidobacteria, with well-researched specifics such as L. rhamnosus and L. casei, so look for these on the label.
- A good supplement has billions, not millions, of bacteria, so again, check the label.
- Probiotics taken in the evening can work well overnight, aiding immune modulation and helping address the root causes of gas.

When you first take a probiotic, the changes within your gut environment may release more toxins and produce more gas in the bowel to begin with. You might feel worse before you feel better, so make sure you eat plenty of vegetables, drink the herbal teas recommended above and rest – it should pass within 3–4 days and you can also take the digestive enzymes below to help your gut cope.

Other digestive and liver supplements

- Consider taking 1–2 digestive enzyme capsules with the first mouthfuls of each meal for a few months to break down the food you eat. Doing this will enhance your body's digestion by reducing stress hormones.
- Magnesium supplements (see page 55) can help release spasm or seizure in gut muscles which can lead either to constipation or diarrhoea, particularly when chronic stress leaves the smooth muscle of the gut struggling to normalize bowel movements.
- Milk thistle (200–300mg daily), is a herb with a long traditional (and well-researched) use for liver support; you may prefer to look for a liver-support blend at your healthfood shop which might include other herbs such as dandelion and artichoke.
- Other gut-healing and supporting supplements might include turmeric as an anti-inflammatory and liver support and glutathione to feed gut cells and as our main antioxidant enzyme.
- Aloe vera juice can help constipation, but do not take it for longer than three months at a time or the bowel can start to rely on it. Take as directed or 2 tablespoons pure liquid on an empty stomach morning and evening. Aloe juice can also be taken with turmeric or crushed fennel seeds to prevent tummy pains.

Delivering soothing, healing and regulating properties to the gut wall

Soothing the ENS through diet includes the stress-coping and blood sugar balance advice given before in relation to other parts of the nervous system. The healthy fats, proteins and nutrients mentioned in previous chapters for brain support are also used for healing and regrowth of the gut wall. Here we add in some specifics for the health of the mucosal lining, the gut environment and to aid our ability to bring down the inflammation related to mood issues that can originate in the gut.

Soups and stews for easy digestion

When it comes to hydrating the gut wall, there is no better way than through soups and stews, and this also includes curries. Soups and stews are low maintenance, can be made in batches for freezing or portioning into dinners and convenient lunches to take to work in a thermos flask. This one-pot approach was man's first cooking method (probably since about 290,000 years ago) and was how we supported our digestion to be able to grow bigger brains, because the fire provides the energy needed for digestion, rather than our own body. Slow-cooking replicates this really well, because by this method nutrients are kept most intact and plant fibres that are difficult for humans to break down are rendered less gas-producing.

There are many different soups and stews in this book and all have plenty of ingredients that contain the minerals and natural sugars that best deliver water into cells, including:

- Spices for gut calming, healing, antioxidants, such as in Spiced Bean Stew (page 94).
- Carotenoid vegetables like carrots and beetroot/beet for fat-soluble antioxidants, such as in Carrot Soup (page 151).

- Coconut milk option for MCT fats (see page 120) for providing fuel to gut wall cells and destroying unwanted invaders like bacteria and yeasts, such as in Thai-style Noodle Soup (page 126).

RECIPES IN OTHER CHAPTERS THAT SUPPORT DIGESTIVE HEALTH

All recipes in this book have some aspect of digestive support – prioritizing vegetables, fibre, healthy fats and protein – and while those that feature in this chapter are specifically tailored to aid the gut, there are some recipes from other chapters that are worth mentioning here for their particularly supportive ingredients:

- Mushroom Pâté (see page 90) – mushrooms are great prebiotic foods and also contain a host of factors that destroy unwanted invaders. Contrary to popular belief they do not feed yeast overgrowths in the gut such as candida albicans (sugar does), but they do have immune-modulating properties, so they help your immune system have an appropriate response (not too much, not too little) via antibodies on the gut wall. This can help dampen down tendencies to inflammation that affect both the gut and the brain.
- Omega-rich Bircher Muesli (page 120) – raw grains in mueslis and other cereals are hard work to digest, can create inflammation on the gut wall and prevent the absorption of key minerals such as iron and zinc. These minerals can be low in a vegan diet, so if you are only eating plants you need to be mindful to eat many more vegetables than grains overall. Breaking down the problematic components in grains – lectins and phytic acid – with processes such as sourdough

fermentation or soaking in an 'acidifier' (such as the yoghurt or apple juice mentioned in the Bircher muesli recipe, page 120) help lessen these issues.

- Smoked Fish Pâté (page 124) – omega 3 fatty acids play an important part in the enormous healing and regrowth of the immense surface of the gut wall. With its finger-like fronds (villi) that help digestion and sense the gut contents, the gut wall is about the size of a squash court and completely regrows every four days!

Fish Soup Provençale

This chunky soup is easy to digest and is high in good-quality protein that helps to balance blood sugar to cope with stress. Garlic is a potent, natural antibiotic while also being antifungal, so it helps to keep the gut environment healthy. Parsley helps calm gases that form as part of digestive processes.

Serves 2–3

1 medium onion, finely chopped

2 cloves garlic, finely chopped

1 teaspoon olive oil

600 ml (1 pint) fish stock

1 tablespoon tomato purée/paste

1 medium courgette/zucchini, finely chopped

15–20 runner beans, finely chopped

1 celery stalk, finely chopped

1 teaspoon dried thyme (or two fresh stalks)

1 teaspoon dried oregano

100 g (3½ oz) white fish, such as haddock or monkfish, cut into cubes

50 g (2 oz) mussels (frozen are probably easiest)

50 g (2 oz) prawns (frozen are probably easiest)

pinch of salt and freshly ground black pepper

1 tablespoon chopped parsley, to serve

1   Soften the onion and garlic in a pan with the olive oil and 2 tablespoons of the fish stock. Add the tomato purée and stir well. Add the courgette, beans, celery, thyme and oregano. Pour in the rest of the stock, season, then cover and leave to simmer for 30 minutes. Add the fish to the soup with the mussels and prawns. Leave to cook for 5 minutes.

2   Once cooked, pick through the soup and discard any unopened mussel shells. Just before serving, sprinkle with the freshly chopped parsley.

3   Note: This recipe can be easily converted to a thicker fish ragoût, or stew, for a heartier dish that serves 4. Simply halve the amount of fish stock to 300 ml (10 fl oz), or 200 ml (6 fl oz) and 100 ml (3½ fl oz) of white wine. Tip in one 400 g (14 oz) can of chopped tomatoes when you add the vegetables to the pan, and add a handful of squid rings along with the fish. Serve with brown rice.

Bean and Courgette Soup

This is a variation on a pistou, or pesto, soup made in France and contains plenty of beans that feed the beneficial gut bacteria. Often because beans give many people gas, this helpful effect comes with discomfort and an extra strain on the liver, but when slow-cooked with onions and garlic the difficult fibres in beans, such as raffinose and stachyose, are much easier to digest.

The pesto that is part of this recipe can also be used as a gut cleanser and detoxification support; it can be served as a side sauce or as a dressing by adding as much olive oil to it as you like.

The Parmesan cheese is optional here, but if you are not vegan, it has an interesting gut benefit. The smell so peculiar to Parmesan is butyric acid (from the Latin word for butter, *butyrum*, where it was first found) that feeds gut cells and is in fact the root cause of the smell of vomit – bringing up all that useful stuff in the gut… But don't let that put you off!

Serves 3–4

1 medium onion, sliced	3 cloves garlic
olive oil, for frying and the pesto	bunch of basil
250 g (9 oz) green runner beans, sliced	3 medium tomatoes, peeled and chopped
2 × 420 g (15 oz) cans haricot beans, drained and rinsed	1 tablespoon freshly grated Parmesan cheese (optional)
2 large courgettes/zucchini, sliced	pinch of sea salt and freshly
1 litre (1¾ pints) water	ground black pepper

1   Ideally, put all of the ingredients in a slow cooker (crockpot) and cook on a medium heat for 8 hours. Otherwise, in a large pan, soften the onion in a dessertspoon of olive oil. Add the runner and haricot beans and courgettes and stir for a few minutes. Cover with the water and simmer for about 20 minutes until the vegetables are softened and cooked through.

2   While this is cooking, put the garlic, most of the basil leaves, tomatoes, a tablespoon of grated Parmesan, if using, and a pinch of salt and pepper in a blender, slowly adding about a tablespoon of olive oil to make a pesto sauce.

3   Check the vegetables are well cooked – if the soup is too thick, add a little more water. Just before serving, pour the pesto into the soup and stir well.

4   To serve, ladle into individual bowls, grate some more Parmesan over each if you like and top with a basil leaf.

Chunky Vegetable Soup

This bog-standard winter veggie soup can be made vegan-style with vegetable stock or cubes, or if you eat meat you can either buy good-quality pre-made chicken stock or make your own from a leftover chicken carcass. The cabbage provides the amino acid (protein building block) glutamine that feeds gut cells, and if you include chicken stock, this is an even richer source – hence the 'Jewish medicine' of chicken and vegetable soup. You can vary the veg here; any cruciferous vegetables (cabbage, broccoli, kale, etc.) provide sulphurophanes, chemicals we use for cell and liver detoxification enzymes, and also provide sulphur for collagen production – for healing the gut wall and other tissues. Squash provides bulk as a potato alternative and also antioxidants in the form of coumarins.

Serves 3

1 teaspoon olive oil
2 onions, chopped
2 carrots, peeled and sliced
2 celery stalks, sliced
1 leek, trimmed and sliced
½ small squash
5–6 kale or Savoy cabbage
    leaves, tough ends removed

3–4 sprigs of fresh thyme
½ teaspoon dried mixed herbs
1 tablespoon rolled oats (if you
    can tolerate them)
1 litre (1¾ pint) vegetable stock,
    home-made or from a cube
pinch of salt and freshly ground
    black pepper

1   Heat the olive oil in a large saucepan and add the vegetables one by one, onions first. Stir well, adding the herbs. Stir in the oats and pour the stock into the pan, adding the salt and freshly ground black pepper. Leave to simmer for at least 45 minutes or cook on a low heat in a slow cooker for 8 hours.
2   Either serve as it is – a rough veggie soup – or put in a blender for a smoother soup.

Bitters and Artichoke Salad

This salad is a wonderful example of a common starter or appetizer around the world. It mixes various 'bitters', which in traditional cultures have long been used to prompt stomach acid production and bile flow for appetite and digestion; hence being served at the beginning of a meal.

Here we use bitter leaves, artichokes and lemon, but other bitter foods are grapefruit and other citrus, olives, ginger, pepper, cardamon, broccoli and other cruciferous veg and culinary spices such as thyme, marjoram, lovage, rosemary, tarragon, bay leaves, sorrel and sage. The herb milk thistle (see page 150) is an example of how bitters also prompt detoxification.

Including as many bitter foods as possible in your diet can counter any reliance on sweet, bland food, but their strong taste can take a bit of getting used to if you haven't been having many, so acclimatize your taste buds slowly.

Serves 2

2 large handfuls of bitter salad leaves

Creamy Vinaigrette (see page 31)

6 artichoke hearts, sliced

4–6 slices preserved lemons, roughly chopped

handful of hazelnuts, roughly chopped

I   Tear the salad leaves into a large bowl, toss in half of the dressing and arrange on the plates. Put the artichokes on top of the salad along with the preserved lemons. Sprinkle over the hazelnuts, then drizzle with the remaining vinaigrette and serve immediately.

Puy Lentil Salad

French Puy lentils make a delicious salad and a great starchy alternative to grains, which many people find harder to digest – even non-gluten types such as rice. It is also good to have variety to hand and the higher protein content of lentils work well for vegetarians. Quinoa would work here, too.

Adding a stick of the seaweed kombu reduces the gas-producing properties of beans; add a large strip of dried kombu seaweed to the pot of beans and water prior to boiling. Remove the kombu once cooking is finished. This is an alternative to slow-cooking pulses in onions and garlic to break down the fibres (see page 156).

This recipe uses basil, but you can, if you prefer, use parsley or even fresh coriander/cilantro. You can use more herbs, too, if the taste suits you; the aromatic oils that give them their pungent smell are warming to the digestive tract and aid its function, and also help expel gas. The abundance of olive oil is soothing and anti-inflammatory to the gut wall, and the lemon juice helps digestion – lemon juice in water has been drunk as a digestive aid since Roman times for good reason. As well as being a bitter food, lemon is known as a cholegenic, as it stimulates bile flow from the liver to enable us to digest fats and regulate the reproductive hormones oestrogen, progesterone and testosterone, which both women and men have in differing amounts and are deeply related to our mood (see Chapter 8). The atomic structure of lemon juice is similar to the digestive juices found in the stomach, so it tricks the liver into producing bile, which helps keep food moving smoothly through your body and gastrointestinal tract.

Serves 2

1 mug of Puy lentils

1 kombu stick (available from healthfood shops)

3 tomatoes

3 spring onions/scallions, finely sliced

6 basil leaves, roughly torn

2 tablespoons cold-pressed olive oil

1 dessertspoon freshly squeezed lemon juice

pinch of salt and freshly ground black pepper

1 Wash the lentils thoroughly in a sieve/fine-mesh strainer set under running water, then tip them into a large pan of cold water with the kombu stick. Bring to the boil and simmer until the lentils are cooked. This should take about 30 minutes – taste to check that they are not hard. Drain and leave to cool, discarding the kombu.

2 While the lentils are cooking, you can pop the tomatoes into the pan for a minute to loosen the skins. Take them out, peel them and chop them roughly. Toss the lentils well with all the other ingredients. I prefer to serve this salad slightly warm, but it is just as good cold.

Grilled/Broiled Mackerel on a Bed of Stinging Nettles

This omega-3-rich fish recipe includes nettles for kidney cleansing, which helps to support the liver as they take on some of its burden and helping process waste products from proteins – nettle tea also does the trick. You can use rocket/arugula here instead if you can't find nettles or be brave, put on a pair of gloves and pick just the tender leaves at the tips.

The chillies here don't irritate the gut as you might expect, actually it's a substance called capsaicin that creates the hot sensation and some evidence suggests it can help with digestion by signalling the stomach to release more digestive juices.

Serves 4

5 red chillies

1 clove garlic

handful of a mixture of sage, thyme and parsley

3 tablespoons olive oil, plus extra for the nettles

4 mackerel, gutted, head on

25 stinging-nettle tips

splash of balsamic vinegar

4 slices of lemon

1   Preheat the grill/broiler. Mash 1 chilli, the garlic and the herbs with the olive oil in a pestle and mortar. Place this mixture inside the fish and secure with a cocktail stick. Cook the nettles in a steamer until they lose their sting – this takes about 5 minutes.

2   While steaming the nettles, put the mackerel under a hot grill/broiler for 3–4 minutes per side – really fresh fish can be left slightly underdone. Toss the nettles in olive oil and lay them on the plates. Put a fish on top of each bed of nettles and splash on some balsamic vinegar. Garnish with a slice of lemon and a whole chilli.

3   Note: If you cannot steam the nettles, just rinse them in water and put them in a saucepan to cook like spinach. Drain the nettles, reserving the liquid to drink later, as it cleanses the digestive system.

Tabouleh

This is a variation on the traditional Lebanese tabouleh, using quinoa instead of bulgur wheat to make a non-gluten version that is kind to the gut wall while also providing protein and oils, as quinoa is a seed, not a grain. Parsley and mint have traditionally been used for digestive function, calming the gut wall and helping to relieve indigestion and flatulence. Parsley is also diuretic, easing water retention and bloating.

Serves 2–3

3 level tablespoons quinoa

6 tablespoons water

1 large bunch of parsley, finely chopped

3 sprigs fresh mint, finely chopped

3 spring onions/scallions, finely sliced

3 medium tomatoes, roughly chopped, plus 1 sliced tomato, to serve

3 tablespoons olive oil

1 tablespoon lemon juice

pinch of sea salt

lettuce leaves, to serve

1   Rinse the quinoa thoroughly in a sieve/fine-mesh strainer set under running water – if it is not rinsed well, it can be bitter. Tip it into a saucepan with the water. Bring to the boil, cover, then simmer until cooked – about 15 minutes. Leave to cool.

2   Once cool, mix the quinoa with the chopped parsley, mint, spring onions, tomatoes, olive oil, lemon juice and salt. Taste to see if you prefer it a bit more lemony. Arrange on a large serving plate surrounded by crisp lettuce leaves and serve with slices of tomato.

Which lifestyle changes best support your digestive health?

Good digestion needs a calm nervous system, so all of the previous lifestyle advice applies to supporting communication through the gut-brain axis. Some specifics can help you connect to your gut, where you have a chance to quieten a busy head.

Mindful eating

We've already mentioned the importance of chewing for digestion, but you can vastly improve the whole process by taking time to relax and enjoy your food, resting for at least 10 minutes after you have finished eating. Slowing down to eat mindfully allows you to feel the full sensations and tastes of your food, and has been shown to help us naturally regulate portion size and appetite. Eating in a state of stress results in food often being only partially chewed, adding to digestive issues. The other positive beneficial effect of chewing is jaw release, unravelling the tight jaw that is common with chronic stress that keeps the mind racing and tension in the gut.

Have periods of digestive rest

In the pursuit of blood sugar balance, the advice is often given to eat 'little and often', but constantly putting things into our mouths starts the whole digestive process from the start, which is both very energy-consuming and gives the gut little time to be empty, which it needs for full healing and motility (moving food through). Eating fully satisfying meals and snacking only when needed (see page 24) also allows you to connect with true hunger, which we will discuss more in the next chapter.

Freeing the organs

Our digestive organs need to be able to move fully, and stress tends to constrict their motion and affect digestion. Doing movements that allow visceral 'slide-and-glide', where the organs can move freely across each other, also helps release trauma that we store down in the belly. Walking – particularly in nature – on uneven ground, naturally prompts these abdominal movements, as well as undulating movements in yoga and Pilates, dancing, t'ai chi and also belly dancing and hula-hooping!

TOP TIPS FOR SOOTHING BELLY STRESS

To optimize your digestion and detoxification, on top of previous chapters' advice, try to:

- Include plenty of vegetables for fibre and prebiotics, especially sulphur-rich cruciferous veg.
- Reduce toxic elements in your life to lessen the burden on your liver.
- Have fermented foods regularly.
- Rehydrate between meals, including with supportive herbal teas.
- Consider a probiotic and other digestive and liver supplements.
- Eat soups and stews.
- Include calming herbs in your diet.
- Take time to eat and chew well.
- Avoid continual eating and snacking too much between meals.
- Move your belly area to free the tissues there, including regular walking.

Part Six
RECIPES FOR FULL SATISFACTION

CHAPTER 6
APPETITE REGULATION

It's all very well knowing what you 'should' be doing, but what about when your good intentions feel constantly derailed by overwhelming and often very sudden urges to eat volumes of the 'bad' stuff? For most people, in this agitated state, what you feel you need to soothe yourself and feel normal is probably not the healthy choice you had planned. More often it is that heady combination of sugar and fat that draws us to self-soothe when our own calming mechanisms are inaccessible.

Increasing numbers of people – especially young women – are reporting that their appetite and eating patterns are out of control. Some people can open a packet of chocolate biscuits, take a couple and put the packet away. For others, this is inconceivable – they cannot resist the urge to eat the whole packet in one sitting, often just to be rid of the constant pull or thought that those biscuits are temptingly close in the cupboard!

Food cravings and overeating are often linked to mood-regulation issues such as depression, anxiety, SAD and PMS, as well as states of loneliness, worry or boredom. It is no coincidence that people tend to comfort eat when they are feeling low, for certain foods trigger chemical reactions in the body that bring some temporary relief. The danger is that occasional comfort eating can turn into a destructive pattern of regular, compulsive overeating that is notoriously hard to break.

In fact, comfort eating, for some people can lead to periods of uncontrolled bingeing which can add to the very stress that contributes to out-of-control patterns, as they are so often accompanied by feelings of guilt and shame – both of which we feel acutely in the body, so that we then turn to food to numb this pain. These cycles are not easy to break as they are a heady combination of biochemistry and psychological survival strategies gone awry.

On the list below, tick the symptoms that are familiar and persistent for you:

- Feeling that your eating is 'out of control'.
- Recurrent episodes of binge-eating.
- Eating large amounts of food quickly, even when not feeling hungry.
- Hiding food (or evidence such as wrappers).
- Eating until you feel uncomfortably full.
- Feelings of disgust or guilt during and after overeating.
- Binge-eating triggered by uncomfortable feelings such as anger, anxiety or shame.
- Disgust or embarrassment about body size.
- Feelings of worthlessness.
- Mood swings and irritability.

If you ticked five or more of the above symptoms, you may be suffering from disturbed eating patterns.

Why do I feel this way?

Whatever the extent of your eating habits, a person of any age, sex or size may suffer from compulsive overeating. Statistics show that many people who experience binge-eating have a history of depression, and that 30 per cent of the women who seek help for weight loss are suffering from this. For those who suffer compulsive overeating as a deeper condition, this may be referred to or even diagnosed by a doctor as binge-eating disorder (BED); this is characterized by frequent episodes of uncontrolled overeating. Unlike bulimics, BED sufferers do not purge themselves after bingeing, and therefore tend to put on weight.

Helpfully, we have covered many of the underlying causes behind disordered appetite signals in previous chapters, but we will delve a little deeper here to add in some specifics for when urges are more persistent. Whether you find this a constant issue or in the form of cyclical compulsions, such as just before periods or in times of work deadlines, there are many factors at play.

Dieting appears to cause a sense of deprivation – as well as starvation and low blood sugar – which can easily result in bingeing, although others find that intermittent fasting (not eating for shorter periods, such as half a day to a day) can help regulate urges. Starting with breakfast as a foundation for the day ahead can help you truly gauge your needs and responses.

The blood sugar balance connection

When bingeing is on very sweet, refined carbohydrates or large amounts of starch (such as pasta or pizza), blood sugar levels rise very rapidly. When your blood sugar drops again, so does your mood – as we explored in Chapter 1. The measures in that chapter are therefore foundational to maintain even blood sugar levels and prevent uncontrollable urges to eat.

These craving cycles may also cause weight gain that can lower self-esteem and feed into habits of bingeing and/or overeating, increasing the likelihood of excess weight, which has been shown to contribute to depression.

The stress connection

Stress, and mostly our reactions to it, is a key player in the overeating cycle. Stress hormones create highs of excitement followed by lows of depletion, and in these dips we can feel a primal need to either dampen intense emotional feelings or shock ourselves out of the torpor of a slump. Humans have been self-medicating through food as long as we have been eating it, we just have more chemicals and processed varieties at our disposal now, and if junk or refined foods were a feature of our childhood diets, our personal brain chemistry will have developed with these substances present and so may struggle to normalize without them. Supporting brain chemistry through blood sugar balance, stress coping and neurotransmitter regulation can help create new patterns and also provide the framework to explore underlying causes through psychological and trauma work, such as talking therapies, with a focus on body awareness and acceptance work (see the end of this chapter).

Excess levels of the stress hormone cortisol is also linked to weight gain, especially around the waist, which can add to feelings of worthlessness that feed into numbing with food.

The neurotransmitter connection

Part of the definition of an addictive substance is one that results in withdrawal symptoms when it is removed and bingeing cycles with changes in brain chemistry; all of this means that the 'addictive' substance creates the feeling of 'normalizing' when ingested. Addictive cycles are more easily formed when brains are in 'famine states' for the substances they need to fully function: the nutrients and blood sugar balance discussed in previous chapters. Without these present, our brains crave the sudden surges of neurotransmitters like dopamine and serotonin that sugar and stimulants can provoke.

When there are inconsistent levels of these neurotransmitters, coupled with sugar lows and disordered cortisol cycles from constant stress, anxiety states can be a side-effect of a body struggling to regulate energy and reacting with an over-excitatory response.

Dopamine is known to be released from the adrenals and nervous system tissue by naturally rewarding experiences such as exercise, food, sex and certain 'leisure' drugs. Dopamine levels can elevate in the presence of caffeine, alcohol and sugar. The way dopamine is used by the brain has been shown to be altered in those tending to anxiety. Many researchers believe that those who suffer from anxiety have a more heightened response to these substances – they get a bigger 'high' – which may result in sensitivity and addiction to substances that create this dopamine release.

Serotonin and carb cravings

As with many disorders linked to mood, people who eat compulsively have also been found to have low levels of the feel-good neurotransmitter serotonin. This can be seen clearly in those who also suffer from some level of SAD (see page 118) and find the winter blues accompanied by overeating or bingeing, particularly carbohydrate (starch and sugar) cravings.

Serotonin is in part responsible for determining our appetite – when serotonin levels are low, we feel more hungry. Carbohydrate-rich foods trigger the production of serotonin, so those (often unconsciously) reaching for more bread, pasta, cereal, cakes, sweets and other starchy foods are self-medicating to regulate mood and boost energy. As we will explore in the recipes, there is nothing wrong with eating starchy foods to improve your mood, as long as you are also considering the fats and protein that you need, especially in winter. It is very sugary, refined foods, such as biscuits, doughnuts and sweets, that are best avoided as these are likely to stimulate weight gain and increase cravings.

Some research has shown that people with SAD who eat more carbohydrates also respond better to light therapy (see page 119), so combining a light treatment with methods designed to increase serotonin levels may be the most effective way of alleviating overeating and/or winter depression.

You are more likely to crave sweet or starchy foods such as chocolate, biscuits or bread if either or both dopamine or serotonin levels are low. These foods indirectly raise serotonin supply to the brain by enhancing the absorption of tryptophan into the brain (see page 81–2), the amino acid that can be converted in the body to serotonin. However, eating very sweet, refined foods is a short-term fix, not a long-term solution. Although they may give you temporary satisfaction, the speedy processing of such foods by the body leaves you craving more soon afterwards (see cravings, page 14). In these situations it is much better to eat unrefined, naturally high-fibre carbohydrates – such as an oat bar, wholegrain crackers with houmous, or fruit with yoghurt. See page 81 for a list of foods that boost your serotonin levels and therefore help to prevent you from craving sweet, starchy foods when you are feeling low.

Chocolate: friend or foe?

Anyone with a sweet tooth or compulsive food cravings knows that sometimes nothing but chocolate will do. Chocolate has been scientifically shown to have in-built feel-good factors, including mental stimulants such as caffeine, theobromine and the 'love molecule' (also in roses) phenethylamine or PEA. Research has shown that many women would chose chocolate over sex and men would chose it over a ride in a sports car!

The sugar in chocolate increases blood sugar levels for an instant energy and mood boost. Combined with fat, the sugar is also believed to release endorphins, or feel-good chemicals, in the brain. Chocolate is a source of the energy mineral magnesium, too, low levels of which are linked to premenstrual symptoms. With this mix of effects, it is no surprise that chocolate is tempting – and addictive.

While the high levels of sugar, saturated fats, hydrogenated fats and other additives in chocolate are clearly not desirable for good health in large amounts, there is certainly no harm in having a little chocolate sometimes. The challenge for a person who tends to binge, though, is how to have a little without succumbing to a lot more.

This is where the 'quality over quantity' approach comes in, with chocolate being a key example. Chocolate comes in many forms and the quality ranges, comparable as a freshly squeezed juice is to a sugary flavoured fruit drink. The health benefits of good-quality dark chocolate are really quite impressive, while those of processed, highly sweetened cheap chocolate are pretty much negligible. The cocoa bean that chocolate is made from has actually been shown to have the highest content of antioxidants as polyphenols and flavonoids, even greater than wine and tea. The higher the cacao/cocoa percentage, the higher its protective antioxidant content (see page 116).

Also when you consider the research that shows that 40 g (1½ oz) a day of dark chocolate helps us cope with stress and can also support blood sugar regulation, there is a case for having rather avoiding it. This is helpful information as it means you can allow yourself a small amount of chocolate in order to satisfy the craving and feel it is helping, rather than hindering, efforts to change habits.

So paying more for higher-quality chocolate and eating less of it can help you become a connoisseur rather than a guzzler, and the same can be said of wine, coffee or any treat. Small amounts of minimally processed plain chocolate with at least a 70 per cent cocoa content contains the most powerful antioxidants and the least amount of sugar, providing the most benefits of plain chocolate you can get. Varieties that provide the best health benefits are:

- Plain chocolate flavoured with mint, orange oil, coconut, chilli, cardamom or other spices as it has the added antioxidant, gut-soothing and blood-sugar-balancing components that these bring.
- Five or six plain chocolate-covered Brazil (or other) nuts as they have more protein from the nuts so come with more flavour and satisfaction.
- Raw chocolate has become popular because, unlike commercial preparation, the beans aren't roasted, retaining much higher levels of antioxidants, a less agitating caffeine effect and are often made with coconut cream instead of dairy.

Addiction or craving?

There's a fine line between what is nutritionally designated a habit and when it becomes an addiction. The labels don't really matter, the point is to observe and be honest about your relationship with what you crave, without self-judgement. And that's not always easy!

If you have addictive patterns with other substances, such as drinking caffeine beyond a couple of cups a day, alcohol, cigarettes, recreational drugs or even behaviours such as shopping, gambling or sex, addressing those also involves blood sugar balance, adrenal (stress support) and neurotransmitter nourishment.

For many, stress prompts cravings, and most often a difficulty resisting things that we are addicted to and even

HABITS VERSUS TREATS

For other food and drinks, buying the best quality you can afford in the same way means you also respect the processes that went into producing it and can feel more connected to your food. This picking of treats based on quality, not quantity, helps change your relationship with them. After all, what is the point of a treat that you don't fully enjoy?

If you're not clear on the distinction, this can help you to observe the difference between a habit and a treat:

- A treat is an occasional enjoyment of something that gives you pleasure but that you do not feel controlled by. Yes, you deserve it occasionally, but you are aware that ultimately it works against your health goals. This means that you can have a little of it and leave some, even take or leave it and not feel a bodily pull from your brain chemistry to have more. You might feel less able to find these boundaries when under stress or upset, when treats can easily turn into habits.
- A habit is something you eat or drink regularly – every day or few days, even feeling it 'normalizes' you. This may be true of the dark chocolate discussed here, or even one or two cups of caffeine a day when you are reducing your sugar intake. We all have habits in life and can recognize them as such, so we don't need to bring in self-criticism. It's when a habit controls us and moves into uncontrollable or damaging territory that we need to take note.

binge-eating at key times of the day (when serotonin naturally dips), most usually at around 4pm and 9pm. Having some well-chosen snacks to hand to pre-empt these urges can help relieve these and help you to feel more able to resist in the future (see pages 38–9).

Alcohol and overeating

Another example of where our habits can be modified for more awareness and less compulsion is alcohol. As something at the top of the list of the foods, drinks and other substances we are likely to turn to when we are feeling down to stimulate our mood and energy, we know that the effects are never long-lasting or genuinely beneficial.

Alcohol puts a strain on your liver and irritates the lining of your digestive tract, making you more susceptible to gut problems and further liver overload. A high alcohol intake is also linked to depression for other reasons: alcohol is sugary, so you get a sharp spike with binge drinking, followed by a dramatic drop in blood sugar levels, taking with them your mood, energy and concentration. Alcohol also stimulates the release of the stress hormone cortisol, high levels of which have been linked to depression. Drinking too much alcohol can also disrupt your sleep, which is discussed further in the next chapter.

If wine is your treat, a better-quality wine and half as much of it at a time can help you savour it. So, for instance, if you're having wine with dinner, choose sulphate-free – preferably organic – and stick to a small glass. Always drinking alcohol with protein tempers blood sugar spikes, so you can practise stopping before you hit the point where you feel unhealthy or guilty. In this way you can find the line where you can control cravings but not deny yourself, so you don't feel the need to rebel and are moving away from feeling confused or neurotic around food.

Alcohol always affects mood – and that is why we might like it – so if you suffer with mood issues and particularly blood sugar swings and compulsions, it is best to drink as little as possible, or even try to avoid it for a while to see how much better you may feel. Alcohol has an immediate (but not long-term) soothing effect, so reducing your intake might cause some temporary agitation. If you have been drinking a lot and suffer anxiety, reduce the amount you drink slowly ('tapering') and seek professional medical help where needed. Magnesium can also help the weaning-off process, see page 54–5.

Addiction or intolerance?

Another piece of this cravings puzzle is that some people seem to crave foods to which they are intolerant, and in eating these foods they become 'addicted' to them. We need to point out here that intolerance is not the same as allergy. An allergic reaction is immediate, obvious and never changes, being an immune reaction caused by immunoglobulin type E (IgE) antibodies. Intolerances, on the other hand, involve IgG antibodies, which need to clump together (agglutinate) before a reaction occurs. This means that the severity and timing of responses are vastly changeable; you may feel an intolerant reaction up to 3 days after eating a certain food, or be able to handle a small amount or just occasionally – it is when you have it too often or in great quantity that enough antibodies are produced to trigger a reaction.

This makes it very difficult to identify foods we are intolerant to, but as a guide, it is possible that the foods we are sensitive to leave us momentarily feeling better, less depressed or less groggy by having an opiate-like effect. As with all highs, this does not last, leaving us in another slump and craving more. By detecting and eliminating from your diet any foods that you may be addicted to, you may well be able to control your food cravings and stop binge-eating.

The notion that food sensitivities can affect mood is still seen as controversial by some medical professionals. Yet clinical experience clearly shows that when some people eliminate certain foods from their diet, quite simply they feel healthier and happier. You may be experiencing a food intolerance if you regularly feel:

- Food cravings, such as for bread or cheese.
- Lethargy or apathy, particularly after eating.
- Fluid retention (symptoms of which include a puffy face, swollen ankles and daily weight fluctuations).
- Feeling better if you don't eat.
- Unexplained grogginess/fatigue.
- Poor concentration.
- Mood swings.
- Unexplained aching.
- Dark circles under your eyes.
- Irritable bowel syndrome/constipation/mild diarrhoea.

If your cravings seem very specific, for example, wanting bread or pasta, this might lead you to suspect wheat is the draw and it might be worth trying to explore intolerance as part of the craving and mood picture.

Common intolerance triggers

Some aspects of the modern diet we struggle to digest well, either because they have not been around long in the human diet (such as for only a few thousand years, not long enough for a true adaptation), or we eat them in great amounts, or they have been genetically modified for human consumption, such as modern wheat crops. Here are the most common culprits:

- Wheat is the most common allergen. If you decide to experiment with avoiding wheat, the following are good alternatives to provide the starchy part of your meal: rye bread (make sure it is pure rye flour); other flour breads, such as rice/soy; rice cakes; oat cakes; rye crackers; oatmeal porridge; oats and other grain breakfast cereals; corn/rice/vegetable pasta; rice noodles; brown rice; quinoa; corn; potato; sweet potato; polenta; millet.

- Gluten: a sticky protein that is difficult for us to digest, this is mostly found in wheat, but also rye and barley and may be in oats that are processed in factories that also make wheat products, so always check the packet for information and warnings.
- Dairy products: designed for non-human baby animals, many of us lose the ability to digest lactose (milk sugar) past early childhood – milk, cheese, ice cream, yoghurt, anything else made with milk – but goat's and sheep's milk is more easily digested by humans.
- Soy: difficult to digest unless consumed in traditional Asian fermented forms; many people become intolerant when they swap dairy for soy and then eat or drink loads without addressing the underlying digestive issues.
- Mould/yeast: found on/in nuts, cheeses, dried fruit, mushrooms, sourdough, beer, and so on.
- Corn and corn products (such as corn oil, starch).
- Food additives and preservatives: notably MSG (monosodium glutamate, added to many processed foods and, most notoriously, much Chinese food).
- Eggs.
- Chocolate.

To detect and address any food sensitivities you may have, assess which foods you eat daily and which you crave – it can be anything, not just from the list above. Eliminate these from your diet, choosing good alternatives (ideally with the help of a healthcare practitioner) to ensure you are not missing out on important nutrients. Introduce each in slowly (at least 4–5 days apart), noticing if your pulse races on eating and up to several hours later. Doing an IgG blood test can be an easier way of determining food intolerance; these are available online or through a nutritional therapist.

Identifying foods we are intolerant to does not address the underlying reasons why these intolerances develop. Supporting the gut wall and full digestion through the measures outlined in Chapter 5 are crucial for preventing and alleviating intolerance. Unlike allergies, intolerances can be changed by removing them and then healing the gut. This includes full chewing of food and even digestive enzymes to ensure partially digested particles of food are not reaching the bloodstream, where they are seen as invaders and set off reactions.

HELPFUL ADVICE ON REGULATING APPETITE FROM OTHER CHAPTERS

- Fats soothe the brain and satisfy the appetite without setting off cycles of craving. Low-fat diets can leave you hungry and constantly wanting to satiate your body's needs. Going for a pseudo-healthy option marketed as zero calories but laden with sugar (such as frozen yoghurt) is not the answer. That can keep you in craving cycles and justifying unhelpful choices – backed up by clever marketing strategies! See the best healthy fat choices on pages 114–15.

- Supporting a healthy microbiome or beneficial gut bacteria can reduce sensitivity on the gut wall and food intolerances that feed into cravings (see page 180–1). This then helps to modulate responses in the enteric nervous system in the gut that allows us to self-soothe more easily, so that we don't need to turn to food to self-medicate.

- Optimizing liver function has been shown to help support weight-loss programmes. It may also support good digestion and blood sugar balance which in turn can help reduce sugar cravings and regulate appetite, as well as supporting digestive and immune function.

- Bitter substances reduce our appetite for sweets and curb a vicious cycle. Sweet flavours prompt the body to distribute more insulin and whet the appetite for more. Wean yourself off a diet based on sweeter tastes and try to get used to more bitter ones (see page 159).
- Supplements for balancing blood sugar (page 22), omega 3 oils (page 112), magnesium (page 55), adrenal support (pages 53–7) and probiotics (page 149) all help to regulate disordered appetite via the underlying causes. You can also look at nutrients needed for sleep in the next chapter if your cravings go hand-in-hand with insomnia issues.

Paying attention to the nourishment we are putting into our bodies can be the difference between setting up yet more cravings and settling our sense of 'enough'. Overeating and compulsive eating lack this sense of satiety, where appetite signals are switched off in the brain. The recipes here add to those in previous chapters to focus on satisfying and soothing the agitated brain chemistry that wants more.

Poached Eggs
with Asparagus

Eggs are protein-rich and a rich source of B vitamins and zinc, all of which help to satisfy the appetite, especially with the fats in the butter and Parmesan cheese, if dairy suits you. Butter and Parmesan can often be better tolerated as both are low in the milk sugar lactose that often causes intolerance reactions.

Asparagus is a great source of inulin, a prebiotic fibre that feeds the gut cells, where many appetite signals begin. It is well-researched that low probiotic levels are related to weight gain and appetite dysregulation. Fibre also helps to satisfy appetite as it provides bulk and stretches the digestive tract, which sends us signals that we are full. Getting this effect from vegetables rather than loads of starchy carbs can help curb the high insulin response that can lead to yet more cravings and weight gain around the middle.

Serves 2

20 asparagus spears
4 eggs
large knob of butter (organic if
    possible)

Parmesan cheese
freshly ground black pepper

1   Trim the asparagus spears and steam them for 5–10 minutes, or until they are tender right through, without allowing them to become too soggy.

2   Meanwhile, bring a pan of water to the boil. To poach the eggs, crack each one into a cup and gently slide it into the water, one at a time, then stir the water quickly to create a whirlpool around the egg. After 3–4 minutes, remove the egg with a slotted spoon. (Alternatively, crack the egg into a ladle and hold it in the boiling water.) Place the asparagus in bundles on two plates and dot with butter.

3   Lay two of the poached eggs on each asparagus bundle and shave a little Parmesan over the top before sprinkling with black pepper. Serve with hot, buttered rye toast.

BAKED POTATO TOPPINGS

For those deep in the throes of low-mood sugar-craving cycles, using starchy carbohydrates such as potatoes or sweet potatoes to stage the sugar comedown is advised. This is a protocol as outlined by Dr Kathleen Desmaisons in her book *Potatoes Not Prozac,* and has proved to be helpful, in particular for those who can resist sugar for three days before a serotonin lull prompts an intense desire for sugar.

The idea is that if your 'need' for sugar is sated by a helping of starches, you'll crave less later on. This is best done at lunch when you'll use the starchy energy for activity in the afternoon, particularly if you want to lose weight. Always having a protein-rich topping such as one of the examples opposite, helps temper any blood sugar rush as the insides of potatoes are pretty high GI (see page 21) – eating the fibrous skin helps to reduce this, too.

To cook your potatoes, preheat the oven to 180°C/350°F/ Gas Mark 4. Wash and prick the potatoes and put them into the oven on a baking sheet for about an hour, depending on the size of the potato; sweet potatoes take less time. Check whether they are cooked through and soft by pricking them with a skewer. Serve them with a Proper Green Salad (see page 32).

Each topping serves 2.

Houmous, Avocado and Seedy Topping

This vegan option mixes the proteins and fats of houmous and seeds with the rich monounsaturate satisfaction of avocado.

4 tablespoons houmous (bought from the supermarket)
½ ripe avocado

2 handfuls of seeds (see page 38 for suggestions)

I   Mash the houmous with the avocado and top with a handful of seeds.

Mustard Chicken Topping

For non-veggies this is a denser protein alternative,
which you may need in times of strong cravings, such
as in periods of stress or with PMS (see page 242).

2 cooked chicken breasts, diced

2 tablespoons plain yoghurt

1 teaspoon wholegrain mustard

freshly ground black pepper

shredded watercress, rocket/
arugula or herbs, to serve

1   Mix the cooked chicken in a bowl with the yoghurt, mustard and
    black pepper. Top with the watercress, rocket or herbs.

Smooth Salmon Topping

The protein and omega 3 fats in salmon support the soothing of brain chemistry. Dill is calming to the nervous system – its name comes from the Old Norse 'to soothe' – and lemon helps the digestion to register 'full' through the gut-brain axis.

200 g (7 oz) wild smoked salmon
1 tablespoon soft goat's cheese
1 spring onion/scallion, finely sliced

1 tablespoon chopped dill
squeeze of lemon juice
freshly ground black pepper

1   Put the smoked salmon into a food processor with the goat's cheese and all the other ingredients and blitz until well blended and smooth.

Roasted Vegetable Salad

The starchy root vegetables here can help calm a raging appetite. The natural sweetness of these veg satisfies any cravings for something stodgy, and helps move trytophan into the brain to be converted into mood-regulating serotonin. This can make a meal that has a protein part or can simply be eaten as a snack without the protein; for those needing a serotonin boost, eating the natural sugars without the protein allows a better uptake of the trytophan moving round in the bloodstream from a previous meal.

Serves 2

1 medium sweet potato (preferably the variety with orange flesh)

1 red pepper, deseeded

1 medium beetroot/beet (pre-cooked, or peel and roast a fresh one yourself)

olive oil, for drizzling

balsamic vinegar, to taste

2 handfuls of lettuce, rocket/arugula or mixed salad leaves

pinch of salt and freshly ground black pepper

1   Preheat the oven to 180°C/350°F/Gas Mark 4.

2   Wash all the vegetables and peel off any bits you don't like the look of from the sweet potato. I tend to leave most of the skin on. Slice the potato into pieces of roughly the same thickness and about 3 cm (1 inch) in diameter. Chop the pepper to the same size.

3   Pour a little olive oil over the sweet potato and pepper pieces in a roasting pan and roast in the oven for 30–40 minutes, or until tender and a little crispy around the edges. Chop up the pre-cooked beetroot into cubes and add to the roasted vegetables – you can warm this through in the oven or let the heat of the cooked vegetables warm the beetroot a little. Season and add balsamic vinegar to taste. Serve warm on the salad leaves.

Warm Caper Salsa

A salsa is simply a cold, spicy sauce of Latin origin, often made with tomatoes and chillies. We've left the chillies out here, but you can add them in to taste. The capers and lime offer a tart kick that wakes up the brain to register the food you are eating, rather than letting you simply eat mindlessly and lose the signals of satiety. Being able to cook this recipe makes simple dishes of protein and veg more exciting, and means you are more likely to cook healthy food from scratch rather than default to takeaways or processed food that you are craving. Serve as an accompaniment to meat, fish, salads or cheese and crackers.

Serves 4

3 small shallots, finely chopped

1 teaspoon olive oil

2 large tomatoes, peeled, deseeded and chopped

1 tablespoon capers

juice of 1 lime

1   Heat the shallots in the olive oil in a small saucepan. When the shallots are soft (do not allow them to brown) add the chopped tomatoes, capers and lime juice and stir the mixture for just a couple of minutes as it warms through.

Japanese-style Tofu Salad

This dish will leave you feeling remarkably satisfied,
yet lightly fed, as is the case with most Japanese food.
This is because of the rich mix of flavours, including the
juxtaposition of bitter, sour, sweet and salty, as well as
the savoury 'umami' taste that we also find in gravy, yeast
extract, cooked meats, mushrooms and cheese. The tamari
provides that here, without the gluten of other soy sauces.
Whether you suspect gluten intolerance or not, it is good
to have the least you can in your diet if you tend towards
overeating – it is difficult to digest and so puts a strain
on the gut, and some research has shown that it affects
serotonin on the gut wall, which is believed to be
involved in appetite regulation.

Visit the Japanese section of healthfood shops for other
flavourings and condiments. Here we've used tofu as the
protein, but you could also use fish, seafood or meat.

Serves 2

350 g (12 oz) firm tofu, cut into
bite-size chunks

large bunch of rocket/arugula

½ large cucumber, sliced into
long strips

4 spring onions/scallions, finely
sliced

8 cherry tomatoes, halved

1 tablespoon sesame seeds,
toasted (black, if possible)

For the marinade

2 tablespoons tamari (gluten-
free soy sauce)

1 tablespoon sake/sherry

½ teaspoon wasabi paste

For the dressing

1 tablespoon lime juice

2 tablespoons tamari or soy
  sauce

2 teaspoons sesame oil

1   First make the marinade. Mix the tamari, sake or sherry and
    wasabi together in a bowl. Add the tofu to the marinade and stir
    to coat.

2   Combine the ingredients for the dressing in a small bowl. Pile
    the rocket, cucumber strips, spring onions and tomatoes on
    two plates.

3   Heat a griddle pan (or non-stick frying pan) and toss the tofu
    pieces for a few seconds on each side to sear them. Lay them on
    top of the salad and drizzle with the dressing. Scatter over the
    toasted sesame seeds and serve.

Kebabs

Kebabs are a wonderful way of eating vegetables with a crunch alongside the firm textures of mushroom, tofu, halloumi or fish to get that sense of satisfaction from the bite and the chew. You'll see there are a few alternatives offered here for the base ingredients and also for a few different marinades, so that you can vary this dish to ring the changes and see which flavours are most satisfying for your taste buds and brain.

Serves 4

2 courgettes/zucchini, sliced crossways

1 red pepper, deseeded and cut into 2½ cm (1 inch) pieces

1 yellow pepper, deseeded and cut into 2½ cm (1 inch) pieces

1 fennel bulb, cut into 2½ cm (1 inch) pieces

4 bamboo skewers

Vegetarian version add:

Portobello mushrooms

Firm tofu or halloumi chunks

Fish version add a variety of seafood such as:

Monkfish

Salmon

Scallops

Large prawns

For the marinade:

juice of 3 limes

3 tablespoons olive oil

1 teaspoon turmeric

½ teaspoon ground coriander

1 teaspoon Tabasco sauce

pinch of salt and freshly ground black pepper

sprigs of fresh parsley, to garnish

1   Cut the mushroom, tofu, halloumi or fish into equal-size cubes. In a large dish, combine all the marinade ingredients and add the mushroom, tofu or fish that you are using, coating them well. Leave them to stand, ideally for an hour. Do not marinate the halloumi. Meanwhile, if you are using wooden skewers soak them in cold water to prevent them burning.

2   Preheat the grill/broiler. Prepare the skewers, separating each piece of mushroom, tofu, halloumi or fish with the vegetables. Grill/broil the kebabs until the fish is cooked, if using, or the other ingredients turn nicely brown – this should take no longer than 12 minutes. Halfway through cooking, turn and baste the skewers with the remainder of the marinade.

3   Serve on a bed of rice garnished with parsley and accompanied by a large green salad.

For a more Western Mediterranean-style marinade

3 tablespoons olive oil
juice of 2 lemons
1 teaspoon chopped thyme
8 large basil leaves, roughly torn

pinch of salt and freshly ground black pepper
a few capers, to garnish

For an Indian-style marinade

150 g (6 oz) plain yoghurt
1 teaspoon ground coriander
½ teaspoon ground cumin
½ teaspoon turmeric

½ onion, grated
pinch of salt and freshly ground black pepper

For a Far Eastern-style marinade

1 tablespoon sesame oil
juice of 3 limes
2 red chillies, finely chopped
2 cloves garlic, crushed

1 tablespoon fish sauce
2½ cm (1 inch) piece of fresh root ginger, grated

Cardamom Oranges

Citrus fruits leave us feeling refreshed, and as a fruit they make one of the best sweet treats that also delivers a satisfying amount of fibre and even protein in the pith. In fact, oranges were the highest-ranked fruit on the 'satiety index', a list of 38 foods put together by Australian researchers in order of how full they left people feeling for the longest time after eating. Oranges were also ranked almost as high as porridge and higher than eggs, bread, pasta and rice. They were an astonishing 3–4 times higher in the list than pastries, cakes and doughnuts!

So reaching for an orange (apples are good, too) is a great first choice when sugar cravings hit. If they then persist, you can reassess, but having this contingency and allowing yourself some time to feel the settling of satisfaction can give you a very viable strategy to unravel the vicious cycle of cravings.

This recipe adds a little more sugar for a halfway house between the simple, unfettered and more healthy fruit and the treat of a 'proper' dessert. It is great to offer at dinner parties to show how healthy choices can be delicious.

Serves 4

3 large or 4 medium oranges

5–7 cardamom pods

3 mugs of water

1 cinnamon stick

1 tablespoon honey or coconut sugar

juice of 1 lime

1   With a vegetable peeler, take a 12 cm (5 inch) strip from the orange peel then cut off the remaining peel and white pith with a knife. Cut the oranges into slices across the middle (so you get a star-shape) and place these in a bowl.

2   Grind the cardamom pods with a pestle and mortar or grinder attachment on a blender, to get enough powdered spice for about half a teaspoon. In a saucepan, bring the water to the boil with the cardamom, cinnamon stick and honey or coconut sugar. Turn down to a simmer, then after 10 minutes, add the lime juice. Turn the heat down to low and simmer until the mixture is reduced to 1 mug, about 50 minutes. Cool the syrup for 10 minutes.

3   Strain, discarding the solids. Pour the warm syrup over the oranges and chill for at least 6 hours or overnight.

Which lifestyle changes best help regulate your appetite?

Appetite issues and cravings are common features of any mood issues, intricately caught up in our mental health in so many ways. Adding to the stress and lifestyle considerations of previous chapters, which will also work for appetite, the next chapter on sleep can also help you to notice how your food wants and compulsions are always tied in to how you are living your life. The more you can bring awareness to your craving responses to when stress rises or when you feel emotionally low, the more choice you have to feel in control of, not controlled by, food.

Appetite control

The body has natural impulses that signal hunger and satisfaction with a meal. However, in some people this messaging system is ignored or becomes unbalanced, often as a result of chronic stress or trauma. One hormone in particular – cholecystokinin (CCK) – aids the digestive process to give the sign that you are full after a certain amount of food. However, partly as a result of extreme over- or undereating, people who binge appear to have either low levels of CCK or a dulled response to it.

It is very important to sit down to eat, then eat slowly and chew well. CCK is released as food enters the small intestine from the stomach. If you eat slowly (see page 140), the hormone is released and the satiety message is received while you are still eating. If, on the other hand, you wolf down your food, the satiety message is not passed on until you have finished eating, by which time it is too late to receive the signal that you have eaten enough.

Natural dopamine highs

When dopamine is low and we feel demotivated, our brains will try to do whatever they can to raise it. When we are not creating enough dopamine of our own, we try to source it via sugar and stimulants. Dopamine is the reward neurotransmitter, it gives us a 'happy' feeling whenever we do anything that propagates the species, such as activities that keep us able to breed well and connected to others, as social animals. This means that exercise, laughter, joy, hugging, singing, eating together, healthy sex and good conversation all help to reduce our need to turn to food as self-medication.

Eating socially when you can also creates more positive associations and connection with the act of eating. If you are a sociable person but live alone, this can affect your desire to be soothed by food. Finding friends to have regular meals with can help you notice this association with food and bring the joy and connection that we need. We are pack animals and can often feel low when we don't have the support of a 'tribe'.

Being in your body

The more we listen to our bodies, the more we can be responsive to our feelings of intuition, rather than simply react to knee-jerk feelings of hurt or want. The more we can be aware of our physical self, in the here and now (known as embodied awareness), the more we can follow intentions to look after our whole being.

We tend to give more credit to thinking than feeling in our culture, and all of this living in our heads can leave us feeling less grounded and less safe. The brain panics when it is not aware of what the body is doing, because it is so vital to be fully aware of our surroundings and our position for our survival responses.

It is a key feature of mindfulness (page 131) to invite the mind to join the body, present in the here and now, to have a full sense of self and feel grounded. This helps to soothe the brain and lessen the continual seeking of the next thing that can be part of stress and hypervigilance, as discussed in Chapter 2. Mindful movement – where you pay kind attention to the subtleties of body sensations – is particularly helpful for a mind used to flitting around and struggling to tether to the body and present moment. Yoga, Feldenkrais, T'ai chi, Qigong and primal movement all offer this support when taught with an emphasis on breath and feeling bodily sensations.

Exploring the root causes

In addressing any kind of compulsive eating disorder, the most successful results are achieved through a combination of psychological and physiological approaches. That is, the patient examines and deals with the emotions that trigger overeating and takes nutritional measures to curb the cravings. For more on talking therapies that can help you to resolve the emotional problems behind your disturbed eating patterns, see page 281–2.

TOP TIPS FOR REGULATING YOUR APPETITE

In addition to advice from previous chapters:

- Have a quality over quantity approach to treats and recognize the habits that you may use to self-medicate.
- Have plain chocolate as an 'allowed' treat that supports the changes you want to make.
- Assess your relationship with alcohol and perhaps have a period of avoidance, if needed.
- Ensure there is plenty of fibre in your diet so that you feel fuller and to support gut bacteria for appetite regulation.
- Use starchy vegetables like potatoes, beetroot/beets and carrots to satisfy signals for a rise in serotonin.
- Use plenty of interesting and lively tastes to register excitement in your brain at the food you have eaten.
- If you are craving sweet foods, try eating an orange or apple first and pay attention to when you register satisfaction at their tastes and textures.
- Explore foods you may be intolerant to, or have an IgG blood test to investigate.
- Slow down to eat and register the reception of your food.
- Explore where you need more connection and joy in your life for serotonin and dopamine levels.
- Practise mindful movement to nurture more connection and acceptance of your body.
- Consider a talking therapy, if appropriate.

Part Seven

RECIPES FOR QUALITY SLEEP

CHAPTER 7
SLEEP SUPPORT

This sleep chapter comes late in the book, but this in no way reflects the important role it plays for our mood and mental health. We have mentioned sleep throughout and have been building up to this all-important recovery phase, as the quality of nutrition and energy regulation throughout the day can greatly determine the quality of our sleep.

You don't have to have full-on insomnia to need to support your sleep. Quality time as well as quantity in the unconscious realms is one of our most important mood factors. Waking feeling unrefreshed, groggy or needing a huge amount of sleep are signs that your time there isn't reaching the full cycles of restoration that you need.

You've probably noticed that your mood, stress-coping and cravings are greatly affected by how much sleep you get, so nutritional support for getting to sleep and staying asleep is a key part of this puzzle.

On the list below, tick the symptoms that are familiar and persistent for you:

- Difficulty getting to sleep.
- Waking up in the night.
- Waking early and not getting back to sleep.
- Feeling unrefreshed after a night's sleep.

- Putting off going to bed, even when tired.
- Energy slumps/dozing during the day.
- Falling asleep early in the evening but not sleeping well through the night.

If you ticked four or more symptoms, you could probably benefit from altering your diet and lifestyle in order to improve the quality and amount of sleep you are getting.

Why do I feel this way?

Ideally we are asleep for roughly a third of our lives. This is not wasted time, but the period where we drop into the parasympathetic nervous system zone – the opposite of the fight-or-flight sympathetic (see page 45) – where we heal, renew, rebuild, detoxify and the immune system can clear up the day's invaders and create new antibodies.

Insomnia (or sleeplessness) can be a symptom of chronic anxiety, depression or stress rather than the cause, and it can often be helped when the other problems are addressed. Whether this is Type 1 insomnia (difficulty falling asleep), or Type 2 (waking in the night), following the recommendations for blood sugar balance, neurotransmitter support and other measures for mental health will help your ability to find and sustain fully restful sleep that allows you to feel calm and coherent during the day. You can also visit your doctor or other healthcare practitioner, or contact an organization that specializes in sleep problems.

Sleep issues can often be a result of our habits and not prioritizing the full relaxation we need in the evening. If we don't respect our need for quality sleep, we are more likely to experience fatigue, irritability, poor concentration and poor recovery from stress, injury and skin complaints. An ongoing sleeplessness problem can affect productivity and relationships. Without adequate sleep, the body quickly shows clear signs of stress and even keeps up the stress response to provide the energy not available without adequate rest. Sleep deprivation makes us tired, moody and irritable and, in the long term, even depressed. Sleep-deprived individuals have also been found to have a reduction in the immune cells needed to resist invaders, reducing their ability to fight off illness and infection.

Your brain is only around 3 per cent of your body weight but it uses around a quarter of your energy, requiring lots of recovery time. Without this it can struggle to regulate and cope with stimuli coming in. We can tend to suffer more anxiety and agitation when we don't get the sleep we need. Our brain processes what the day and life has thrown it when we are in REM sleep (see below) – when the brain is more active than when we are awake – and whether we remember our dreams or not, we need this inner reflection for a psyche that can settle and make sense of what it finds.

Understanding your sleep cycles

Sleep is a state of altered consciousness, where we drop into brain cycles where we have a relatively low sensory relationship with the external world. Nearly all of our voluntary muscles – the ones we can control to move around – are inhibited and we move between two distinct states: REM (Rapid Eye Movement) and non-REM sleep.

During both waking and sleeping, our brains run through 90-minute cycles; these are similar, but obviously the night-time ones involve dropping down deeper into unconsciousness. During sleep there are four stages of non-REM sleep (about 75 per cent of the night), followed by REM, which gets longer each time throughout the night, with the longest period lasting an hour.

Non-REM stages:

- Stage 1 – between being awake and falling asleep; if you wake here you can feel like you weren't asleep. This lasts about 5–10 minutes.
- Stage 2 – light sleep where the heart slows and temperature drops to prepare us for deep sleep. Here we disengage from our surroundings and our breathing becomes irregular.
- Stages 3 and 4 – deep sleep phases, with 4 being the deepest; here brainwaves slow down (delta waves), blood pressure drops, muscles fully relax and the blood supply to them increases. This is where tissue growth and repair happens. Hormones for growth and development are released and energy stores are replenished. This is where restoration occurs.

REM (25 per cent of night):

- First occurs about 90 minutes after falling asleep and is then reached every 90 minutes – the brain is active dreaming, but the body is immobilized (muscles switched off) to stop us acting out our dreams as if they were real, although the face, fingers and legs may twitch. This state gives the body energy and has a correlation with how well we can perform during the day.

REM sleep is unique to mammals and uses up more energy than when we are awake. Non-REM sleep uses 11–40 per cent less, so this is when we rest and recover. In REM, some researchers believe that the quick eye motions are not following what we see in dreams but are an external manifestation of memory processing. REM is where we dream; emotion centres in the brain light up in this state, whereas they dampen down during non-REM.

The first two complete sleep cycles are thought to contain mostly sleep of Stages 3 and 4; REM (dream sleep) occurs mainly in the second half of the sleep period; and lighter sleep (Stages 1 and 2) comes only at the end of the night. If you are deprived of sleep for a while, at the earliest opportunity your body will try to make up this deficit by quickly going to Stage 4 and REM sleep in each cycle.

Stress and sleep

Many of our body's daily rhythms, including those that dictate our energy and sleepiness, are finely tuned mechanisms that depend on certain hormonal patterns, body chemicals and nutrients. At night time, levels of the hormone cortisol should dip, calming your body and preparing it for sleep. If, however, your cortisol levels are out of kilter for any reason (usually owing to stress or a diet high in stimulants or sugar), your ability to get to sleep, to sleep through the night or to wake up refreshed is likely to be impaired. If cortisol levels are high at night, this suppresses the release of growth hormones, which are essential for daily tissue repair and growth.

Stress taken into the evening can not only keep you awake, it can also increase the likelihood of your body laying down fat, especially if you eat late, too. Evening relaxation helps keep your appetite appropriate for the low level of activity that your body expects at night, and helps your digestion at a time when it is slowing down. A nutritional therapist can arrange a laboratory saliva test for you to determine whether your cortisol rhythm is out of synch. See pages 51–2 for dietary advice on supporting your adrenals and regulating cortisol production.

Sleep in the modern world

Our body clocks – that is, the 24-hour daily metabolic rhythms set into our biochemistry – have been in place from when we lived in caves. They follow the light-dark cycles of the sun but continue even when we don't see daylight. This means ideally waking on sunrise and going to bed at sunset, obviously not something your average twenty-first-century dweller is doing. Simply putting lights on when it is dark outside, or watching TV and surfing the net disrupt this system, which is naturally designed to shut you down for rest and recovery. Our ancestors would have wound down by socializing with the tribe, chatting, eating, dancing and, of course, having sex!

Chronic tiredness at night is common, and often comes about because of physical difficulties in dealing with stress during the day. After a day of commuting, looking after children, working 8–18 hours with no lunch break and evenings spent texting or surfing the net, it's understandable that we feel exhausted at the end of the day. Slumping on the sofa watching TV is not an ideal recipe for sleep, as the flickering lights and constant moving imagery keeps our brains in a stressed state, even when our bodies seem to refuse to move. This is why the nutritional and lifestyle support for the daytime in previous chapters is so crucial; sustaining energy and mood throughout the day allows us to have the motivation in the evening to choose active relaxation (see pages 131–2) so that we can gently and enjoyably allow our nervous system to quieten down ready for full sleep.

Sleep and blood sugar balance

Balancing blood sugar levels in the daytime means we have the energy to exercise and bring down stress hormones at night so that we don't have any nervous, unused energy when it's time to sleep. Blood sugar highs and lows during the day also set

MAGNESIUM AND GABA OVER ALCOHOL

Much like sugar hits shoot up energy in the short-term only, alcohol has the illusion of a quick-fix 'cure' for sleeplessness. This effect is produced by stimulating the neurotransmitter GABA (gamma-aminobutyric acid), which decreases excess adrenaline, calming the nervous system and switching off a chatty mind. We should be able to produce this naturally around bedtime, but we need the mineral magnesium to do so but many of us receive too little in our diets (from green leafy vegetables, fish, nuts and seeds) while using it up quickly through stress, as it is a relaxant in its own right. Taking a magnesium glycinate supplement (300–400mg) with dinner may help support quality sleep.

GABA is produced by our brains in response to alcohol, cannabis or tranquillizers and many turn to these to help switch off at night. However, the effects are short-lived and if these are taken close to bedtime, the comedown can disturb REM sleep, as ultimately they reduce our ability to respond to our own natural production. The following foods also help us produce GABA: bananas, broccoli, citrus fruits, white fish, nuts and legumes. Meditation and yoga have also been shown to raise GABA, without the come-down, so these are better evening choices!

up waking-in-the-night tendencies (particularly when it can drop suddenly around 3–4am); if we can't sustain even levels during the day, we are on a steep downward trajectory when we go to bed. This means we can hit a low before morning and this hypoglycaemia prompts a release of adrenaline to prevent us dropping into a low blood sugar coma. This is when we can wake suddenly in the small hours of the night with sudden worries, fears or even thinking something is in the room or house, as we are waking to this immediate stress-fear hypervigilant response where our senses are suddenly ramped up on alert.

The following habits that throw out blood sugar levels and cortisol also affect sleep:

- Skipping breakfast and then playing 'catch-up' all day for sustained energy. This means that you are more likely to snack or eat later in the day, with digestive processes going on at a time when your body should be directing energy towards building up, healing and renewal, rather than breaking down food.
- Late-night sugar bingeing providing quick-release energy that prevents the nervous system dropping into calm states, often as a result of dropping serotonin levels. (See the previous chapter.)
- Excessive caffeine during the day or for those sensitive to it, beyond 2–4pm.
- Late cigarette smoking: like the other stimulants above, this raises cortisol levels. If you are a smoker, consider a plan to stop and at least avoid smoking from early evening onwards.

The serotonin–sleep link

Serotonin (see pages 81–2) has a central role in sleep-cycle regulation, so basing a light supper around tryptophan-containing foods – such as bananas, chicken, milk, sunflower seeds, tuna, turkey and yoghurt – from which we produce it can help to promote sleep. Serotonin levels rise to calm us down in the evening and then we produce the sleep hormone melatonin from serotonin, which governs our circadian rhythm. Melatonin is also an important antioxidant, one of the reasons why getting enough sleep is anti-ageing.

Having a carbohydrate snack before bed has the double whammy of providing a source of sustainable sugar throughout the night to help prevent sudden waking, and provoking production of the hormone insulin to take these sugars into cells for energy. Insulin is needed to move trytophan into the brain and low levels of serotonin signal sugar cravings for this effect. Late-evening carb cravings and binges are linked to this mechanism (see last chapter), so try to choose something that will help rather than hinder sleep. Grandma's 'biscuit by the bedside' is not the 'perfect' nutritional solution, but it has some credence. A halfway point like a small flapjack or oat-based biscuit may be the answer if you are really craving sugar while you make changes that help you move towards healthier choices, such as:

- Oat or rice cakes with houmous or goat's cheese or a slice of chicken or turkey.
- Oat or rice cakes with tahini and a little honey or nut butter.
- A small pot of plain yoghurt with sunflower seeds/chopped dates or figs/bananas.
- Banana milkshake (with coconut or almond milk).
- Piece of fruit and a handful of sunflower seeds or almonds.
- A couple of dried dates and a few sunflower seeds or almonds.

Avoiding stimulating foods

If you feel agitated in the evening or struggle to get to sleep, it may be worth eliminating foods that are high in tyramine. This amino acid (protein building block) increases the release of norepinephrine, a brain stimulant that interferes with the ability of the nervous system to calm and move towards sleep states. Foods that contain tyramine include chocolate, aubergine/eggplant, potatoes, sauerkraut, sugar, processed (such as smoked or cured) meats and fish, tomatoes and red wine. Essentially anything aged, dried, fermented, salted, smoked or pickled can be high in tyramine, so if you struggle with sleep, it may be a good idea to save the sourdough bread, sauerkraut and Parmesan for breakfast or lunch!

Nutrients for sleep

We have mentioned the calming mineral magnesium many times as one of the most important nutrients for mood, energy, self-soothing and also sleep. As well as increasing levels through diet (see pages 54–5) and reducing the factors that use it up quickly – stress and sugar – in order to break a cycle of daytime anxiety leading into night-time sleep issues, supplementing magnesium at night and even in the morning too, may provide great relief.

Magnesium works with B vitamins, so ensuring you are getting adequate amounts through your food and a supplement if needed (see page 55) helps support mood and energy regulation that leads into healthy sleep, as well as your ability to deal with stress. Take a B-complex early in the day rather than in the evening as they are energizing.

- Magnesium glycinate is a form that can help produce sleep neurotransmitters in the evening, see more information in Chapter 2.
- Vitamin B6 is the only B vitamin recommended at night. Others can stimulate, but B6 is needed to produce GABA and serotonin and works with magnesium. A supplement up to 50–100mg can be taken with dinner. You should stop taking it if any numbness or tingling occurs, but this is extremely rare.
- If you have long-term insomnia you may also find a supplementation of 500–1,000mg of the amino acid

taurine helpful alongside magnesium, and it is often found in calm or sleep supplement formulas. Taurine is found in fish, meat and milk, so vegetarians may need to supplement it; the body can produce some but this may suffer in times of stress or low vitamin B6 levels. Taurine and magnesium act like GABA, our brain's natural 'braking system', to help us switch off and fall asleep. This may be particularly helpful if overthinking or recurrent thoughts are getting in the way of sleep.

- Also see the amino acid L-theanine on page 56, which can be taken in the morning to help anxiety and at night to help sleep (100–200mg each dose), all part of the same pattern of self-soothing capacity.

Many sleep supplements will contain these nutrients and maybe also the herbs mentioned below.

For women: the cycle of sleeplessness

Many women find that how long and how deeply they sleep varies with their menstrual cycle; sleeplessness is particularly common just before a period or during the menopause. Because oestrogen influences the production of brain chemicals that keep you alert, and progesterone can trigger sleepiness, it is not surprising that hormonal fluctuations cause sleep variations. Supporting hormone regulation can also help sleep; it is no coincidence that nutrients involved there (see pages 249–51), such as vitamin B6 and magnesium, can also help with sleep difficulties.

The Gut-Brain Axis

Going back to the information in Chapter 5, it is useful to know that the gut goes through a similar 90-minute cycle to the brain. They evolved together in humans as an organism and within you personally, in your embryological growth in the womb. Many people with digestive issues also experience sleep issues and can see mood linked to both. Supporting the regularity of your gut motions can feed into the quality of your sleep.

Natural sedatives

Sleep aids of any kind are unlikely to provide much benefit if there are other underlying factors that are keeping you awake at night. If you're eating badly, drinking a lot of coffee or alcohol or are particularly stressed, you need to resolve those issues first in order to give any natural remedies the best chance to work.

Medical sedatives are generally bad news in that they are usually addictive. As your tolerance of them increases, you need to take ever higher doses to feel any effect. They can trigger a range of side-effects, including daytime drowsiness, memory problems, confusion, depression, dry mouth, sluggishness and all sorts of other unpleasant symptoms. Medical sedatives are also strong chemicals that need to be detoxified by the body, placing a burden on your liver.

There are many non-addictive natural substances that can help you sleep, although they should be used only occasionally.

- Drinking chamomile tea or sleep teas that include this herb help to keep us asleep by raising levels of the neurotransmitter glycine. This is effective not just before bed but has an accumulative effect when chamomile is regularly ingested, reducing anxiety and allowing us to sleep through the night.
- Valerian, hops, passionflower, oats and lemon balm (melissa)

are all herbs that have a long history of use as sedatives and are also often found in sleep tea formulas, but they can also be taken medicinally.

- A couple of drops of lavender on your pillow is soothing and can help lull you to sleep.
- See other foods covered in the book that soothe the nervous system and are traditionally known as sleep, as well as anti-anxiety, remedies, with research to back them up – such as celery, lettuce (page 189) and dill (page 53).

Your eating rhythms determine blood sugar and digestion. You are more likely to sleep well if you eat your main meal at lunchtime and have a lighter meal in the early evening; eating slowly and in moderation allows full digestion. If your body is busy digesting a recent meal, your sleep will be disturbed, and if you are suffering indigestion, bloating or gas, the discomfort this causes can worsen that. If you can, eat at least three hours before going to bed and if you do need a small bedtime snack to sustain energy through the night (see page 213), also eat that while sitting, slowly and consciously.

Observing our food habits through the day can have a great effect on our sleep that night, and certain food choices can have an even greater impact.

Filling Fruit Bowl

This simple recipe can be a good breakfast choice for those not used to having a full, or even any, breakfast. Weaning yourself onto eating within the hour after you get up can help support blood sugar balance that leads into sustained levels through the night and also supports the adrenals to enable you to fall asleep easily. The seeds blend used here provides protein and fats to help these actions. The fruits in this bowl are less sweet than some, with great fibre content for slow energy release, and the yoghurt and seeds provide trytophan for serotonin production. Even if eaten in the morning, the trytophan can still be moving around in the bloodstream later and regulation throughout the day also supports sleep at night. Seeds (and nuts) also contain the hormone melatonin that we need to fall asleep.

This also makes a great bedtime snack – especially if you tend to late-night sugar cravings – but it is better to choose one of the savoury options if you are watching your weight.

Serves 2

8 tablespoons plain yoghurt or coconut yoghurt

4–6 pieces or servings of fruit from the following list: pear, apple (or even purée), berries (fresh or frozen), plums, apricots, peaches, nectarines, prunes or banana and figs as trytophan sources (prunes and bananas are also good B6 sources)

2 tablespoons ground High-Five Seeds (see page 57)

I   Put the yoghurt into two bowls and pile the fruit on top, chopped into small pieces if necessary. Top each with a heaped tablespoon of ground High-Five Seeds.

Mongettes Charentaises

This is a lovely light evening meal or a side dish for lunch. The word *mongettes* is the local Charente term for white haricot/navy beans and these, or any other beans you like, provide the building blocks for the soothing neurotransmitter GABA. They are also fibre-rich with plenty of prebiotic action, feeding the good gut bacteria we need to regulate neurotransmitters and also provide a sense of satisfaction that can stop the late-night agitation of seeking sugar or starches.

There are tomatoes here, which we mentioned as a stimulatory tyramine food earlier, However, tomatoes also contain melatonin to help sleep, so it is best to gauge how they make you feel in the evening.

This is a dish that is usually made from scratch using dried beans that are soaked and cooked through, but you can also slow-cook, or if simply making them as here, add in the kombu stick as before (page 59) to aid digestibility and alleviate gas before bed. Traditionally the dish is served with roast lamb, making a great meal for meat-eaters and providing a rich source of trytophan to produce sleep-inducing serotonin.

Serves 2, or 4 as a side dish

extra virgin olive oil, for cooking
2 x 400 g (14 oz) cans white
   beans, or fava beans, drained
   and rinsed
1 large onion, chopped
2 large tomatoes, chopped

2 cloves garlic, finely chopped
large sprig of fresh thyme
2 bay leaves
large pinch of sea salt and freshly
   ground black pepper

1 Heat the olive oil in a large heavy saucepan and toss in the beans
   with the onion and tomatoes, stirring for a few minutes until
   the onions are soft, but not brown. Add half a can of water, the
   garlic, thyme, bay leaves, salt and pepper and allow to simmer for
   about 20 minutes.

2 Serve immediately or cool and store in the fridge for later –
   these beans taste great the next day.

Warm Noodle Salad

Eating something as easily digestible as this warming bowl at night reduces the energy needed for the digestion process, which becomes less efficient overnight – the time when we are detoxifying, repairing and rebuilding most. Chicken, tofu and white fish are all great sources of trytophan, but you could also add pieces of ready-made plain omelette instead for the protein element, as eggs are another rich source.

Rice or buckwheat noodles are wheat- and gluten-free starchy carbohydrates, so these are less likely to put a strain on the digestion than wheat noodles (or the egg ones that still contain wheat) tend to, and which can upset sleep. Grains such as rice also contain melatonin, the sleep hormone.

Serves 2

200 g (7 oz) rice or buckwheat noodles

1 tablespoon olive oil

1 clove garlic, crushed

4 baby corn

½ red onion, sliced

1 carrot, peeled and sliced

2 tablespoons white cabbage, shredded

handful of mangetout/snow peas

350 g (12 oz) chicken, tofu or white fish, cut into bite-size pieces

juice of 2 limes

1 dessertspoon sesame oil

1 dessertspoon tamari or soy sauce

1 handful of coriander/cilantro, chopped

1 Cook the noodles according to the packet instructions. Drain, rinse in cold water and place in a serving bowl.

2 Heat the oil in a wok or large pan and add the garlic and a tablespoon of water. Add the vegetables when the garlic is soft (not brown). Toss the vegetables until wilted. Add them to the noodles. Cook the chicken or fish in the wok, stirring until cooked through, or warm through the tofu in the wok. Add these to the noodles. Toss everything together with the lime juice, sesame oil, tamari or soy sauce and coriander.

Grilled/Broiled Rainbow Trout

For those who eat fish, it is an amazing sleep combination of tryptophan, magnesium and vitamin B6. Choosing an oily (and sustainable) fish like trout also provides omega 3 fats. Having higher levels of the omega 3 DHA in your system is associated with better sleep, as it is needed to produce the hormones required to fall asleep – such as melatonin – and also for receptor sites that pick up these and neurotransmitters. Taking fish or algae omega 3 supplements (see page 112) at night rather than in the morning is often recommended for those with sleep issues for this reason.

The chives are a good source of choline, an important B vitamin that helps your body with sleep, learning and memory, as outlined on page 86. We mentioned that taking B vitamins at night is not recommended in supplement form (except B6) as they are energizing, but you do not get this effect from food sources.

If you are intolerant to dairy or simply want a lighter meal, you can grill/broil the trout and add chopped chives with a generous drizzle of olive oil instead of using crème fraîche or yoghurt.

Serves 4

4 rainbow trout fillets, washed and patted dry
200 ml (7 fl oz) crème fraîche or full-fat Greek yoghurt

bunch of chives
100 g (3½ oz) cooked prawns/ shrimps

1   Place the fish fillets under a preheated hot grill/broiler for 2–3 minutes on each side.

2   In a saucepan, heat the crème fraîche or Greek yoghurt along with the chives and prawns, until warmed through.

3   Put each of the rainbow trout fillets on a plate and pour the sauce over them. Serve with a Proper Green Salad (see page 32) and steamed broccoli, or any other veg side dish.

Gobble Pie

This is a healthier version of a traditional meat and potato pie. A vegetarian version can be made using two 200 g (7 oz) cans of aduki, borlotti or other beans instead of turkey, all rich serotonin sources, as are the sesame seeds. We've used sweet potato instead of the usual white to include less quick-release starch and more brain-supporting, fat-soluble nutrients such as beta-carotene that give the orange colour – much more supportive of blood sugar balance throughout the night.

This is a true comfort food, so that rather than turning to big starchy meals, you can get the warming, soothing satisfaction with high nutritional value. There is plenty of fibre here to support digestive and detoxification processes. Research has found that including more prebiotics in our diet that feed our beneficial probiotic gut bacteria means we spend more time in restful and restorative sleep, known as non-rapid-eye-movement (NREM) sleep. This is probably due to the neurotransmitter support that comes from those produced in the gut wall and the signalling back up to the brain that good probiotic levels in the gut ensure.

The inclusion of parsley helps soothe the gut wall and reduce gas build-up in the digestive tract that can interfere with quality of sleep.

Serves 4

500 g (1 lb) potatoes, peeled

1 large onion, chopped

2 cloves garlic, crushed

1 tablespoon olive oil, plus 2 dessertspoons

1 carrot, finely chopped

1 celery stalk, finely chopped

500 g (1 lb) minced/ground turkey

200 g (7 oz) canned tomatoes

2 tablespoons chopped parsley

1 dessertspoon tamari or soy sauce

1 dessertspoon Worcestershire sauce

1 bay leaf

2 dessertspoons sesame seeds

pinch of salt and freshly ground black pepper

1   Put the potatoes into a pan of cold water, bring to the boil, and cook for about 15 minutes until soft.

2   Meanwhile, soften the onion and garlic in 1 tablespoon of olive oil and 2 tablespoons of water in a saucepan. Add the carrot, celery and turkey and stir until the meat is browned. Add the tomatoes, parsley, tamari or soy sauce, Worcestershire sauce and bay leaf and stir well. Cover and leave to simmer. Check every now and then, and add water if it is drying out. When the potatoes are cooked, drain and mash them with 2 dessertspoons of olive oil and season.

3   Preheat the oven to 200°C/400°F/Gas Mark 6. Remove the bay leaf from the turkey mixture and put the meat into an ovenproof casserole dish, keeping back some of the liquid if it is very watery. Season with pepper. Top the meat with the mashed potatoes and sprinkle the sesame seeds on top. Bake for 20–30 minutes, or until the potato is golden brown.

4   Serve with steamed broccoli.

Carrot Soup

Sometimes we feel we can only digest a very light meal in the evening. Soups or stews (such as any in this book) make a great comforting meal before bed.

Carrot provides a rich supply of fibre and brain-protecting beta-carotene. As with many ingredients in the recipes in this book, the vegetables, olive oil, herbs and spices support liver detoxification. Our main detox phase is around 3–4am and sleep may be disrupted around this time when the liver is struggling or has lots to deal with, so these foods can help. The brain has its own unique toxin clearance system, the glymphatic system, which is ten times more active during sleep, effectively clearing wastes and plaques back to the liver for elimination. So both helping sleep and supporting cleansing helps us function during the day on many levels.

The Tabasco and black pepper are optional, as spicy foods may give some people indigestion that interferes with sleep, as is the ginger, but it is worth including as it can calm the gut and relieve gas before bed.

Serves 3

I onion, chopped
I clove garlic, chopped
I teaspoon olive oil
a few sprigs of fresh thyme
½ teaspoon mustard powder
½ teaspoon wild onion seeds
1¼ cm (½ inch) piece of fresh root ginger, grated
2 pinches of salt

dash of Tabasco Sauce (optional)
freshly ground black pepper (optional)
I litre (1¾ pints) chicken or vegetable stock
500 g (1 lb) carrots, peeled and chopped
2 celery stalks, chopped
plain yoghurt, to serve

1 Soften the onion and garlic in a large saucepan with the olive oil and the herbs, spices and flavourings, adding a couple of tablespoons of the stock after a minute or so. After another 4–5 minutes, add the carrots and celery. Stir well. Pour in the rest of the stock, bring to the boil then turn down to a simmer and cover. Leave to cook for about 40 minutes. Add more water if the soup thickens too much.

2 When the ingredients are cooked, transfer the soup to a blender or use a hand blender to blend until smooth. Serve swirled with a teaspoon of yoghurt.

Turmeric and Chamomile Hot Milk

This late-night drink combines the wonderful benefits of chamomile tea (see page 148) with reassuring and relaxing warm milk. It also provides healthy fats from the coconut oil to bulk up those in the almond milk, so it has the soothing effect that a traditional late-night dairy drink can bring. The turmeric and other spices are gut-calming and anti-inflammatory and help your detoxification and immune processes overnight, but do feel free to vary these according to taste and omit any you feel upset your digestion.

There is the option to add honey or maple syrup, but you may find the almond milk, coconut oil and cinnamon sweet enough. You could start with the teaspoon full of sweetener (or more if it helps you to drink this regularly) and then bring the amount down – bit by bit – to acclimatize your palate to less sweet and more subtle tastes.

Serves 2

2 teaspoons turmeric

½ teaspoon ground cinnamon

1½cm (½ inch) piece of fresh root ginger, peeled and grated

¼ teaspoon ground cardamom

½ teaspoon ground nutmeg

2 teaspoons virgin coconut oil

½ mug brewed chamomile tea, warm

1 mug almond milk

1 clove

1 teaspoon good-quality honey or pure maple syrup for vegans (optional)

1   In a mortar, add the turmeric, cinnamon, grated ginger, cardamom, nutmeg and coconut oil and grind with a pestle to form a paste, adding one or two teaspoons of the chamomile tea if you need to loosen it.

2   Heat the almond milk in a pan with the clove until warmed through, then either discard the clove or leave it in to infuse a little longer.

3   There is enough spice paste for two mugs, so you can either share with another or save half for the next night. With half in a mug, pour over half the remaining chamomile tea and half the hot almond milk, warming up more in a saucepan if you need to, then drink while warm.

Which lifestyle changes best help your quality of sleep?

The period of time leading up to going to bed is all-important for the way we sleep, much as the time when we wake sets the tone for the day. We can't always get to bed early, particularly if that involves a mood-enhancing dose of healthy socializing, but it is important to recognize when you need to go to bed early and allow yourself to catch up on sleep. For those who love going out, it might be necessary to evaluate where your social life might be draining rather than recharging you. Does one night out make you feel connected and happy, whereas two in a row leave you having difficulty falling asleep and prone to craving refined carbs the next day?

If you are continually tired or waking unrefreshed, prioritize restful evenings for at least half of your week, or have a 'holiday at home' once a month when you fully focus on sleep quality for a week. This is great for stressful times when your sleep has become affected and you have slipped into those over-stimulating evening habits. Keep a journal if that helps to consider what makes a difference and how you can implement these factors as regular habits.

Soothing towards the end of the day

Our bodies are actually preparing for sleep from 4pm, when they shift metabolism from active to recharging, which is why we can feel a natural lull in energy then. It is a good idea to take a break at this time and allow your energy to increase naturally. Also avoid all stimulants past this time: caffeine, alcohol, sugar and even TV or the computer once you're home from work.

Anything you do at the very end of the day should be moving you towards a calm 'alpha' brain state: baths (see Epsom salts, page 132), reading non-thrilling books, listening to soothing music, doing a calm yoga practice or meditation will ensure quality rest – see more examples of active relaxation on pages 131–2.

Communicate only with people who make you feel comforted and safe, not those who whip you up with difficult emotional issues at a time when you need your brain to relax. This includes phone conversations, well-chosen social media and physical interaction.

Preparing your sleep chamber

Sleep in a chilly and fully dark room. Too much heat or light can halt the production of melatonin, so try to lessen unnatural light wherever possible and use candles if you can. Switch off as many electrical devices in your bedroom as possible. Electro-Magnetic Fields (EMFs) from cordless phones, wireless and mobile-charging hubs can disrupt your sleep quality. If you take a phone to the bedroom, for instance for audio books, switch it to flight mode so no signal or info comes in.

Take care that your bedroom reflects how you would like to live. If it is cluttered, a clear-out could create the space for good-quality sleep. Spend some time creating a safe cave that is to your tastes – even the smallest changes with pictures, ornaments and bedlinen can make you want to spend more time there, enjoying the surroundings as you relax towards sleep. Aim to have as consistent as possible a bedtime and wake-time, to let your body feel safe in its rhythm, and be in bed by 10–11pm as often as possible; the hours before midnight can be more restorative than those after.

Help for waking in the small hours

The brain loves language and if your mind is racing in the wee hours (often 4am, when we are beginning to move towards waking), providing it with alternative voices such as guided meditations or audio books can intercept the hypervigilance coming through as worries, fears or going through those things we know that we need to do. Try not to look at your phone or the time, though!

TOP TIPS FOR QUALITY SLEEP

In addition to advice from previous chapters:

- Sustain energy throughout the day and be ready to bring it down in the evening for quality sleep, including eating breakfast to encourage less late-evening eating.
- Reduce evening stimulation from diet and lifestyle.
- Avoid using alcohol to help you relax or fall asleep.
- Eat foods that help produce GABA and don't eat tyramine-rich foods if you are sensitive to sleep disturbance.
- Ensure you eat plenty of trytophan-rich foods throughout the day and evening.
- Have a snack before bed if you tend to wake in the night.
- Drink soothing bedtime teas or a warm turmeric milk before bed.
- Supplement magnesium in the evening, alongside vitamin B6, taurine and L-theanine if they work for you.
- As often as possible, enjoy calming and soothing evenings to reset your nervous system.
- Prepare your bedroom as the perfect sleep space.
- Use guided meditations or audio books if you wake in the night.

Part Eight

RECIPES FOR HORMONE-BALANCING CAPACITY

CHAPTER 8

BALANCING FEMALE HORMONES

Last, but not least, we come to the – often mysterious – effects that fluctuating or dropping levels of reproductive hormones can orchestrate for many women. Hormones are our body's messengers and can have a great effect on mood, either on a daily basis or at certain times of the month. This can be bound up in stress levels, digestion and liver status and other factors, such as blood sugar balance.

Here we will explore the particular role that female hormones play with mood, focusing mostly on oestrogen and progesterone, the two hormones responsible for the female menstrual cycle and fertility, and whose lowering levels post-menopause can also affect mental health and outlook.

It is worth mentioning that although the advice here focuses on female hormones, many of the nutritional and lifestyle recommendations can apply to men, too, as they also have these hormones present (just in lower amounts); testosterone also can have a huge impact on mood.

On the list below, tick the symptoms that are familiar and persistent for you around your period or generally if you are postmenopausal:

- Chocolate, sugar and carbohydrate cravings.
- Overeating.
- Water retention, puffiness, bloating.
- Mood swings.
- Irritability.
- Despair or a sense of insecurity.
- Feeling tearful or anxious.
- Tender breasts.
- Clumsiness or forgetfulness.
- Excessive tiredness.
- History of hormone-related issues such as endometriosis, fibroids, PCOS (polycystic-ovary syndrome) or breast, cervical or ovarian cancer.
- If menstruating, heavy, painful or irregular periods.
- If perimenopausal, fluctuating periods and moods.
- If postmenopausal, low mood and motivation, and other symptoms.

If you experience any of the above and feel they relate to your monthly rhythms or they did when you were menstruating, if you have stopped, then looking at how your body regulates its sex hormones can be a big part of the mood puzzle. Yes, this obviously changes when we transition into menopause, but the underlying areas that support may still apply if we have kept dietary and lifestyle habits that affect hormones in place – the symptoms or 'expression' may simply be different.

Hormones present for reproduction deplete in the third stage of life; this is a natural process and if you are feeling at odds with this rhythm, understanding some of the factors behind their regulation can help you make effective changes that also ripple through other parts of your life. This may be particularly true of specific conditions such as endometriosis, which is inflammatory and needs anti-inflammatory measures (see pages 116-17), and PCOS is related to stress and sugar.

Within the balance of female hormones, the two main players are oestrogen and progesterone. These act as part of the rhythm of motivation and recovery; oestrogen influences the production of brain chemicals that keep you alert, and progesterone triggers more restful and drowsy states. We can see that they affect mental health both through our ability to feel motivated, but also to sleep and restore brain function. When there is a dominance of one, we can find ourselves and our lives dictated by that, and our mood and health can follow. As an overview, here are some of the many influences of oestrogen and progesterone, showing how they have a see-saw effect with one creating an action that opposes the other:

OESTROGEN	PROGESTERONE
Causes depression, anxiety and headaches*	Acts as a natural antidepressant and calms anxiety
Causes poor sleep patterns*	Promotes normal sleep patterns
Impairs blood sugar control*	Helps normalize blood sugar levels
Increases body fat and weight gain*	Helps use fat for energy
Causes fluid and salt retention*	Acts as natural diuretic
Improves memory	Causes sleepiness, depression**
Improves sleep disorders	Causes digestive problems**
Relieves hot flushes and night sweats in menopause	Precursor of cortisol, the stress hormone
Interferes with thyroid hormone function*	Facilitates thyroid hormone function
Causes cyclical migraines*	Prevents cyclical migraines
Increases risk of blood clots*	Normalizes blood clotting
Reduces oxygen levels in all cells*	Restores proper cell oxygen levels
Seen to cause endometrial cancer*	Prevents endometrial cancer
Increases risk of breast and prostate cancer*	Decreases risk of breast and prostate cancer
Restrains bone loss	Stimulates new bone formation
Reduces vascular tone (dilates blood vessels)*	Improves vascular tone
Triggers autoimmune diseases*	Prevents autoimmune diseases
*Indicates that these effects are caused by an imbalance of oestrogen, caused by too much oestrogen and/or too little progesterone	**Indicates that these effects are caused by an excess of progesterone

You'll see that each has action and limiting effects, but that many health conditions common in modern society may be linked with an excess of oestrogen. This oestrogen dominance may be a result of stress, alcohol or dairy consumption, or hormone disruptors such as plastics and chemical toiletries, and we will explore this further in this chapter.

The need for liver and digestive support

The liver is the heart of hormone regulation. Women produce most of the sex hormones in the ovaries (although some oestrogen is also released from fat cells and some progesterone from the adrenal glands), but the liver plays a vital role in recycling and breaking them down. Addressing the factors that put strain on liver functions and supporting detoxification processes and gut health as outlined in Chapter 5 is foundational to both female and male reproductive health, at any age. For instance, some women – especially those who suffer from irritability, depression and insomnia – see dramatic reductions in their PMS symptoms when they ease the burden on their liver simply by giving up coffee or alcohol.

We need to fully eliminate used hormones (and other substances such as cholesterol) as part of their regulation, so this is yet another way by which good digestion is fundamental to mood health. In particular, constipation can upset hormones as they can be reabsorbed from a stool that is sitting in the colon, rather than being egested. One of the main ways of encouraging your body to eliminate waste optimally is to make sure you are regularly eating naturally fibre-rich foods, such as fresh fruit and vegetables, beans, lentils and whole grains. We can also ensure we have good probiotic bacteria levels in the digestive tract.

Oestrogen circulating round the bloodstream is raised by alcohol, as they have the same liver detoxification pathway.

As alcohol is a neurotoxic (damaging to the brain), our bodies prioritize breaking that down, so oestrogen ready to be detoxified in the liver remains intact. This does not mean that alcohol post-menopause is a good solution for keeping up oestrogen levels! It still strains that liver detoxification pathway, which breaks down a whole host of other substances and depletes vital nutrients.

Other factors that raise oestrogen are dairy, coffee, sugar, smoking, alcohol and stress.

The stress and hormone connection

All hormonal systems in the body are intertwined; your stress hormones and those that regulate blood sugar are not separate to your reproductive hormones. A naturopath or nutritional therapist looks at your adrenal, sex and metabolic (energy-regulating thyroid and pancreas) glands together, to support them all. Particularly when chronic stress is a predominant underlying cause for health issues, supporting the adrenal glands may be the most important factor in sex hormone regulation.

One of the reasons for this is that our steroid hormones all work within the same pathways in the body. These are fat-based hormones that we make from cholesterol, and as well as oestrogen and progesterone, they include testosterone (for men and women), the stress hormone cortisol and aldosterone, a hormone that regulates fluid levels (hence we can bloat when stressed). Cortisol is actually produced from progesterone, so chronic stress tends to lower progesterone and create relatively higher oestrogen levels; another route to oestrogen dominance.

This is why many menstruating women experience heavier periods with shorter cycles (day one to the next day one of a period) when going through times of stress. Oestrogen governs the first half of the menstrual cycle and proliferates the womb lining; with more oestrogen the lining is heavier. Progesterone governs the second half (after ovulation) so if there is less of it, this dominance has a shorter time frame. This can often be a sign you need to look at the demands in your life and support your adrenals, as outlined in Chapter 2. Low progesterone levels have been associated with fatigue and depressive states.

Blood sugar balance and reproductive hormones

As we have established, an imbalance in blood sugar levels is registered as a stressful event for the body and tends to create a responsive rise in cortisol. It also causes surges in glucose and therefore a spike in the hormone insulin which takes glucose into cells for energy. That spike prevents your hormones triggering ovulation, which prevents the signal to produce progesterone, leading to oestrogen dominance.

Sugar also feeds into oestrogen dominance as it leads to the creation of fat cells, and those secrete oestrogen. This is why we need to be a healthy weight post-menopause, because fat cells are the source of oestrogen post-menopause, which prevents bone loss and supports sleep. This is why blood sugar balance throughout the day and month supports mental health on a hormonal level, too. High sugar consumption can often be seen alongside hormonal issues such as PMS, irregular cycles, acne, fertility issues, PCOS and others. Sugar directly leads to inflammation, which is present in endometriosis and PCOS, especially when insulin resistant.

Mood and PMS

PMS (premenstrual syndrome, sometimes referred to as premenstrual tension, or PMT) is an all-too familiar part of their monthly cycle for many women. This slide into misery entails anything from three days to two weeks of mood swings,

NEED AN IRON BOOST?

If you've been having heavy periods and mood issues, it is worth checking your iron levels with your doctor. Low iron levels can show up as tiredness and demotivation through poor oxygenation of blood and lowered production of ATP, our energy 'currency'. You might also experience low mood and sugar cravings, because iron is needed for serotonin production and thyroid function. Vitamin B6 is needed for iron utilization, and vitamin C for absorption, so make sure you have a good intake of these, too. Don't eat iron-rich foods or take iron supplements with calcium supplements, tea or antacids, as these inhibit its absorption.

Food sources

- Animal sources – haem (the form from which we can make haemo-globin in blood): red meats, fish, poultry, organ meats, eggs, dairy.
- Vegetarian sources – non-haem: prunes, dried figs, sesame seeds, tofu, pine nuts, millet, beans, lentils (butter/lima, haricot/navy, pinto, black), spinach, watercress.
- Oats, beans and lentils, soy beans and grains contain non-haem iron, but they need to be prepared to break down substances such as phytic acid. This means soaking oats, as in the Bircher muesli on page 120, slow-cooking beans with garlic and onions, eating traditionally-fermented forms of soy (miso, tofu, tempeh) and grains in bread as sourdough.

How to supplement iron

Normal supplementation range: 4–40mg daily, often found in a multivitamin and multimineral; do not take high amounts without checking levels as this can exacerbate inflammation.

Best forms to supplement: iron bisglycinate (gentle iron), glycine amino acid chelate, ferrous fumarate or gluconate are readily absorbed and cause fewer intestinal side effects.

discomfort and upset. One US study concluded that up to 40 per cent of women who menstruate experience some PMS symptoms. Because it is so common, even extreme symptoms are sometimes dismissed as normal or inevitable, yet most women who suffer from PMS say that it adversely affects their relationships with family and friends.

The primary hormonal disturbance in PMS is the oestrogen dominance discussed above, where oestrogen levels are elevated and progesterone levels are reduced. This can lead to low levels of serotonin as well as impaired liver function, low endorphin levels (pain-relieving substances) that leave the sufferer more sensitive to pain and increased aldosterone secretion, which causes bloating and fluid retention.

In addition, fluctuations in insulin and thyroid and adrenal hormones caused by stress, low nutrient status, caffeine, sugar, saturated fats and little exercise can have a knock-on effect. The fluctuating hormone levels that cause PMS are often not as cut and dry as too much of any one thing, but need an overall regulation of all hormones, including those involved in stress, blood sugar balance and sleep. Having a good look at your particular PMS symptoms can help you to find a starting point for support.

PMS is categorised into four types:

PMS – An oestrogen dominance

- Mood swings
- Irritability
- Anxiety
- Nervous tension
- Sore breasts.

Oestrogen dominance is the most common form of PMS, seen in roughly 76 per cent of sufferers. As we've discussed, stress piled on top of this can cause periods to be even closer together, with some people menstruating every 21–23 days.

Weight gain is usually linked to high oestrogen levels; oestrogen can be stored in fat cells, but it may still not be picked up if the receptor sites are unhealthy or it is not released into the bloodstream, instead it can be stored stubbornly in fat cells. Weight distribution is then normally seen around more 'female' areas – hips, thighs and bottom, the classic 'pear-shape'. The advice for balancing female hormones alongside the use of phytoestrogens (page 248) and liver support (page 150), is to reduce stress and increased exercise, which are vital for all round hormone balance. Low thyroid function and excess weight can also predispose someone towards oestrogen dominance; both need blood sugar support.

PMS – D   Progesterone dominance

- Depression
- Crying spells
- Forgetfulness
- Mild mental confusion and poor concentration
- Insomnia.

Progesterone dominance is much more rare, occurring in roughly 23 per cent of PMS sufferers, although hormones can fluctuate depending on diet, lifestyle issues, stress, emotional and exercise factors. This means that differing types of PMS can be seen on different months and women may experience a variety of symptoms throughout the month according to the highs and lows of oestrogen and progesterone. As with oestrogen dominance, we should concentrate on all-round hormone balance in the same way.

PMS – C   Carbohydrate Intolerance

- Craving for sweets
- Increased appetite
- Fatigue
- Headaches

- Dizziness or fainting
- Heart pounding.

This is linked to poor blood sugar balance affecting oestrogen and progesterone levels, but it also worsens premenstrually as the same nutrients are used to make insulin and female hormones; especially magnesium, zinc and vitamin B6. This means that when production of these hormones is raised, the ability to balance blood sugar can be impaired and more support is needed in that direction.

PMS – H   Aldosterone dominance
- Water retention
- Breast tenderness
- Abdominal bloating
- Weight gain (1.3 kg/3 lb or more).

Aldosterone dominance leads to PMS associated with breast tenderness, fluid retention and general excessive weight gain. There is usually an imbalance of the electrolyte minerals, where sodium is retained and potassium excreted; potassium-rich foods such as celery, almonds and plenty of greens help to address this balance, but dealing with the stress response is also important as it raises aldosterone. Good levels of magnesium (see page 55) are needed to address these imbalances and help cope with stress; a therapeutic dose to help with fluid balance, stress response, proper conversion of hormones and also good sleep quality.

Aldosterone dominance is also associated with prostaglandin imbalances, these are localized hormones that are made from the omega 3 fatty acids and therefore supplementation may help (see page 112). These are also needed for correct oestrogen and progesterone production, and liver function.

NB: When we take hormone medications, our own natural production of these can be reduced, as the body sees there is an external source and then stops making its own. This can happen specifically with the contraceptive pill, which may not have been in harmony with a particular hormone imbalance in the first instance, when prescribed.

Mood in the perimenopause

The timeframe in which a woman's body is preparing to cease menstruating, is around a six-year transition. She may experience many symptoms over this time, the first being changes in regularity and character of her periods – from much shorter and more frequent to the other end of the scale – and these can fluctuate wildly. This confusion is a push-pull between the pituitary gland in the brain and hormones levels in the body. As progesterone and oestrogen are naturally dropping, the pituitary senses that less is available and sends signals to increase production, resulting in wild swings from low to high, and as we've seen with the emotional influences of these and other hormones, this can produce a rollercoaster ride of mood and responses.

All of the support previously mentioned applies here, alongside a recognition that this is a natural time of change and one where fewer demands and more recovery may be needed. This can be great guidance for shifting expectation of how much we can 'get done' on a day-to-day basis and where our true quality of life lies. For example, if sleep is affected, more focus on the nutritional and lifestyle factors outlined in Chapter 7 can help us attune to our new needs.

Mood in the postmenopause

Postmenopause (post- means 'after') is the phase in a woman's life where she no longer menstruates. This time is defined as one calendar year after her last period. Although this signals much lower levels of oestrogen and progesterone, we still secrete oestrogen from fat cells – which is why being

ACTIVE INGREDIENTS: PHYTOESTROGENS

Some plants contain substances known as phytoestrogens ('phyto' means plant), which can help to regulate oestrogen in an adaptogenic way (as do the adrenal adaptogens on pages 55–6), raising that which is too low and lowering that which is too high; and evening out imbalance in the ratio between oestrogen and progesterone.

Phytoestrogens appear to work by locking into the oestrogen-receptor sites on cells – in doing so they block out the stronger human oestrogens or even xenoestrogens from the environment (see pages 260 and 263). At the same time, if a woman is actually low in oestrogen – during the menopause, for example – phytoestrogens act as a weak oestrogen. They thereby help relieve the woman's symptoms by boosting oestrogen levels while still blocking out the harmful xenoestrogens.

It is therefore helpful for women to include phytoestrogens in their diet at any time in their lives. In Asian countries such as Japan and China, phytoestrogens have been long associated with lower breast cancer risk, derived from traditional soy products that are common in the diet such as miso, tofu and tempeh. Soy is a particularly rich source of oestrogen, but fermented forms are best, rather than chemically processed 'modern' versions such as soy milk, textured soy protein (TVP – textured vegetable protein) and soy mince.

Phytoestrogens are also found in citrus fruits, oats, fennel, alfalfa, liquorice, celery, flaxseeds, beans, sesame, rice bran, peas, carrots, apples and pears. Herbs that are good sources of phytoestrogens include sage, parsley and basil.

underweight is a risk for osteoporosis – and progesterone from the adrenals, reminding us that this third stage in life is the time to slow down and enjoy life fully.

This shows how the Goldilocks approach ('not too little, not too much') applies with hormones; while high oestrogen during menstruating years can be associated with depression and irritability, low levels post-menopause are often accompanied by a drop in serotonin, leaving you with feelings of sadness and hopelessness. Oestrogen isn't simply 'bad', it can just tend to be raised before menopause by common modern dietary, lifestyle and environmental factors. Oestrogen also increases GABA, the calming neurotransmitter (see page 211) and raises feel-good endorphins, so we can feel these are compromised – affecting sleep and joy – in later years.

Every woman's experience of the menopause is individual, but mood swings are common, often related to disturbances in sleep and discomfort of other symptoms, such as hot flushes and vaginal dryness. It is crucial to have enough fats in the diet to support this time, as these are critical for hormone production, immunity, brain function and cholesterol metabolism. Low-fat diets can be very harmful as our need for good fats increases with age and stress and women who have been on low-fat diets can find the menopause more problematic, especially mood issues.

Key foods for hormone balance

Like many therapeutic foods, the foods listed here have multifaceted actions that regulate and modulate, rather than simply boost or lower. This is a clever part of nature, as without testing we can never really know what our hormones are up to. Even with testing, though, we can only ever approximate a snapshot of their action at a particular time, especially with blood, a transport mechanism where everything is constantly changing to find homeostasis, or balance. Some foods that we evolved eating (or their modern counterparts) continue to work with our body systems. Because their effects are regulatory, they apply to both female and male hormones:

- Cruciferous vegetables (see page 158) contain sulphur compounds and indole-3-carbinol, which bind to oestrogen and escort it out of the body, reducing oestrogen dominance, which can also affect men and is known to contribute to prostate cancer. Try to eat three servings a day of cabbage, broccoli, kale, pak choi, cauliflower, Brussels sprouts, cavalo nero or mustard greens.
- Citrus fruits contain the antioxidant D-limonene that helps break down oestrogen in the liver – just one portion a day is said to help reduce oestrogen dominance. These fruits can even be blended whole and added to smoothies, because much of the D-limonene is in the peel, but be sure these are organic (this goes for if you use the peel in any way) as pesticides are easily absorbed into the essential oils found there and they act as xenoestrogens.
- Many mushroom varieties contain naturally occurring chemicals that inhibit the enzyme aromatase, which is involved in oestrogen production. This is where they have gained their reputation for lowering the risk of oestrogen-related cancers such as breast cancer, prostate cancer, ovarian cancer and others; as well as weight gain. 'Medicinal mushrooms' are mostly those used in Traditional Chinese Medicine, such as Shiitake, Reishi and Maitake, which contain a type of complex carbohydrate called glucan that balances blood sugar and has been shown to effectively relieve menopausal fatigue.
- Green tea has also been shown to lower oestrogen so well that avoidance in menopause has even been recommended in some camps, although much more research is needed. This

makes it great for those with breast cancer risk or showing signs of oestrogen dominance while still menstruating.

Supportive supplements

As well as blood sugar balance, stress, liver and the digestive measures previously mentioned, you can add in some specific support for female hormones:

- Magnesium appears to work synergistically with vitamin B6 and the mineral zinc for both reproductive and blood sugar balancing hormones. However, many women struggle to convert B6 into its active form and so may benefit from taking this directly as P-5-P (pyridoxal-5-phosphate) rather than the usual pyridoxine in most supplements. As many as 80 per cent of women with PMS have been found to have low supplies of the mineral magnesium.
- The herb Agnus Castus has a long traditional use of regulating periods, from early menstruating years up to perimenopause. It can be recommended by a herbalist or bought in good healthfood shops with the dosage instruction on the label. Stick with it, it can take a few months to work.
- During menopause, several herbs can help the transition to lower hormone levels, but it is best to see a herbalist to ascertain which is right for you; Dong Quai and Black Cohosh are well-researched and used but each has differing effects on oestrogen and progesterone.

The recipes here add in specific hormone-balancing actions on top of any that also support the foundational blood sugar balance, stress-coping capacity and detoxification and digestion support. Every change you make to support your health will ripple throughout your body, as all systems work together, but it is good to also know some tweaks to help your individual needs.

Salmon Rolls

The blood sugar balancing effects of the protein in salmon and the liver-supporting action of its omega 3 fats make this dish the perfect vehicle to add in other hormone-balancing components. The onions provide sulphur for liver detoxification and the soy (tamari is gluten-free) and beansprouts are phytoestrogenic. Cucumber is cooling for those with menopausal hot flushes, but the heat of ginger also supports circulation, essential for delivery of hormones to cells.

Serves 4

4 salmon fillet steaks
1 cucumber, sliced into long thin strips
4–6 spring onions/scallions, sliced into long thin strips
large handful of beansprouts
8–10 tablespoons tamari or soy sauce
2½ cm (1 inch) piece of fresh root ginger, grated
3 tablespoons toasted sesame oil
at least 16 rice pancakes

1   Steam the salmon for 8–10 minutes or poach for about 5 minutes until the fish is cooked through – the flesh should be opaque, not translucent when you cut into it. When it is cooked, break it up into flakes with a fork and leave it to cool in a serving bowl.

2   Arrange the cucumber and spring onions with the beansprouts on a serving plate. Mix the tamari or soy sauce, grated ginger and sesame oil together and divide among two small serving bowls.

3   Prepare the pancakes following the packet instructions.

4   Put the serving dishes onto the table and get people to roll some salmon and vegetables in a pancake (or large lettuce leaf) and, using their hands, dip it into the sauce before eating it. Served with stir-fried vegetables and plain rice, these rolls make a great focus for a dinner party.

Spicy Bean Salad

This very simple and portable lunch is packed with hormone-balancing and detoxifying fibre from the beans, which are also a good source of the bone-supporting mineral boron, especially needed post-menopause. It is vital for bone health as it may prevent calcium being excreted by up to 40 per cent and is also said to double the level of circulating oestrogen in menopausal women. Other examples of boron-rich foods include green leafy vegetables, nuts and non-citrus fruits – especially plums, apples, grapes and pears.

You can use canned beans here, but where possible it is better for your hormones and all aspects of mood support to either soak dried beans overnight or buy them in glass jars – then you are avoiding the toxic metals from the tins that disrupt hormones and agitate the nervous system leaching into the beans. As a staple meal, you can vary the flavours by using one of the dressings described on page 31.

Serves 2

400 g (14 oz) beans, such as pinto, borlotti or mixed
1 large tomato, roughly chopped
2 spring onions/scallions, sliced
10 runner beans, sliced
1 teaspoon soy sauce
1 dessertspoon olive oil
1 tablespoon finely chopped coriander/cilantro
dash of Tabasco sauce (optional)

1   Mix the beans with all the other ingredients and serve.
2   Note: You can use parsley instead of coriander, and freshly ground black pepper instead of Tabasco. Or, for a more Mediterranean version, use lots of olive oil, lemon juice and parsley with a bit of sea salt, leaving out the soy sauce, coriander and Tabasco.

Crunchy Oriental Salad

This is a wonderful combination for hormones; with the cruciferous, detoxifying cabbage, fibre-rich carrot, D-limonene-containing lime and gluten-free soy sauce tamari as a phytoestrogen. The seaweed also supports the thyroid gland as it is rich in the mineral iodine, from which we produce the thyroid hormone thyroxine. Low thyroid function often goes hand-in-hand with female hormone issues, and even if it shows 'normal' on a doctor's test, we can see it still needs support if we feel sluggish, tend to constipation, have difficulty losing weight and struggle to get up in the morning.

Sesame seeds and flaxseeds contain oestrogen-binding lignans, as well as having phytoestrogenic action. Sesame also contains vitamin E to help reduce menopausal hot flushes and antioxidant sesamoid compounds to reduce oestrogen-associated inflammation. It can also be eaten in tahini as a spread on rye bread (also phytoestrogenic) or as part of a dressing, simply mixed with olive oil.

Serves 3

palmful of dried seaweed, such as arame

2 medium carrots, grated

¼ white cabbage, shredded

3 spring onions/scallions, finely sliced

about 10 sprigs of fresh coriander/cilantro, roughly chopped

1 dessertspoon sesame oil

juice of 2 limes

1 tablespoon tamari or soy sauce

1 tablespoon sesame seeds

1   Put the seaweed in a mug, pour on just about enough boiling water to cover and leave to steep.

2   Meanwhile, add the carrots to a large bowl with the white cabbage, spring onion and coriander.

3   Check the seaweed is soft and drain it in a sieve/fine-mesh strainer, tossing it to allow it to cool off before adding it to the salad. Add the sesame oil, lime juice and tamari, and toss all the ingredients together well. Just before serving, sprinkle with the sesame seeds.

Miso and Seaweed Broth with Tempeh

Another Asian dish here, because in cultures such as Japan, the traditional use of fermented soy has seen lower levels of breast cancer risk, although these are now rising as their adoption of Western dietary habits increases. In this take on a Japanese warming bowl (the oldest cooking pottery has been found in Japan), both the miso and tempeh provide phytoestrogens and the seaweed supports thyroid action for adrenal and reproductive organ support. The texture of tempeh is not for everyone, so you can use firm tofu, Shiitake mushrooms, chicken or prawns instead.

This is a more involved recipe, but you can always make a simple miso broth by boiling some water with green veg and adding garlic and ginger, then add any firm tofu, cooked chicken or prawns you want, turn off the heat and add in miso paste to taste (you can buy miso as a paste in a jar for a really quick dish!). You can even add in dried seaweed. Get used to whipping it up quickly so it feels simple to prepare.

Miso bowls can be wonderful warming breakfast alternatives, as they are eaten in Japan, to help you start the day feeling clean and nourished.

Serves 4

200–300 g block of tempeh, sliced into strips, or 1 chicken breast

10–15 g (½ oz) wakame seaweed

1 litre (1¾ pints) water

225 g (8 oz) purple sprouting broccoli (or other green veg of choice)

225 g (8 oz) silken tofu

4 spring onions/scallions, chopped

5 g dulse seaweed

½ teaspoon ground white pepper

¼ teaspoon chilli powder (optional)

4 tablespoons miso paste (brown/white or a mix)

For the marinade

1 teaspoon honey

1 tablespoon mirin

1 tablespoon soy sauce

juice of ½ lime

¼ teaspoon ground white pepper

pinch of chilli powder (optional)

1–2 teaspoons oil

1 To make the marinade, stir together the honey, mirin, soy sauce, lime juice, pepper and chilli, if using, and pour this over the slices of tempeh in a bowl to marinate for anything between 15 minutes and overnight.

2 Preheat the oven to 180°C/350°F/Gas Mark 4. Add the wakame seaweed to a bowl, breaking it up into lengths of around 2.5 cm (1 inch), then pour boiling water over the seaweed and leave to soak for 15 minutes. Place the tempeh on an oiled baking sheet and cook in the oven for 15–20 minutes, 20–25 minutes if you are using chicken. You can check that the chicken is cooked by inserting a knife or a skewer into the breast and checking that the juices run clear (not pink), or cook the tempeh until crisp and browned. Slice the cooked chicken into strips.

3 While the chicken or tempeh cooks, prepare the soup. Drain the wakame seaweed and discard the water that it was soaked

in, as this will be salty. Add 1 litre (1¾ pints) of water to a pan and bring to the boil. Add the broccoli or green veg and wakame seaweed and boil for a few minutes, then add tofu crumbled into about 1 cm (½ inch) chunks along with the spring onions, dulse seaweed, pepper and chilli powder, if using, and simmer for a further few minutes. Add the miso to the pan to heat through but do not boil once the it has been added. Ladle into a bowl and top with chicken or tempeh. Serve hot.

4   Note: You can vary the ingredients in this dish; try adding dried Shiitake mushrooms – you can soak these in hot water for 15 minutes and add the soaking liquor to the broth with the mushrooms at the start of cooking.

5   You can store any extra soup and tempeh in the fridge for 4–5 days and reheat as needed.

Crunchy Carrot Salad

This simple salad is rich in soluble fibre, from the carrots, which is similar to that also found in apples, oats, berries and beans, and which bind to oestrogen in the small intestine to prevent it being absorbed. This reduces your exposure to xenoestrogens from your diet, helping them to be eliminated in a bowel movement. The lemon and the sunflower seeds (you could even increase more!) add to the phytoestrogen potential and you could also add some shredded cabbage for a bigger bowlful and more hormone-balancing action. The olive oil here is also anti-inflammatory, so can help reduce any mood-affecting inflammatory effects of excess oestrogen.

Serves 2

3 medium carrots

3 spring onions/scallions, finely sliced

1 tablespoon olive oil

juice of ½ lemon

1 tablespoon toasted sunflower seeds

1 Grate the carrots and toss together with all the other ingredients. Serve immediately.

Shiitake Roast Chicken

This is a recipe for meat-eaters and uses organic
chicken to reduce the xenoestrogens and hormone-
disrupting growth hormones used in non-organic farming.
Ensure your organic meat is from a good free-range source
and the animal has been able to run around during rearing
(not just for health reasons, but ethical ones, too) and eat a
natural diet for the healthiest omega-rich fat profile. If you
do eat meat, it is best to pay more for this level of quality
and animal welfare, and eat it less often.

This recipe uses shiitake mushrooms, which are prized for
their hormone-balancing and immune-modulating (see
page 250) qualities, as well as their ability to
support the adrenals.

Serves 4

1½ kg (3 lb 5 oz) whole chicken
4–6 cloves garlic, sliced
lengthways
2–3 whole cloves garlic
4 tablespoons tamari

1 lemon
8–12 dried shiitake mushrooms
freshly ground black pepper
2 teaspoons honey
1 mug of boiling water

1   Preheat the oven to 190°C/375°F/Gas Mark 5.
2   Place the chicken in a roasting tin/pan. Use a sharp knife to make
    incisions in the breasts and fleshy legs of the bird and insert
    the garlic slices into the slits. Put the whole garlic cloves in the
    bottom of the roasting pan. Pour in the tamari and rub it all over
    the bird. Cut the lemon in half and squeeze the juice all over the
    outside of the chicken. Then slice one of the squeezed lemon
    halves into three and lay the pieces over the top of the chicken.
    Place the other lemon half inside the cavity. Arrange the shiitake

mushrooms around the chicken and grind black pepper all over. Add the honey to a mug of boiling water and stir well so that it dissolves completely. Pour this mixture into the bottom of the roasting pan.

3   Roast the chicken in the oven for about I hour I5 minutes, or until the juices between the leg and the body run clear when pierced with a sharp knife. Baste the meat every 20 minutes during cooking.

4   Serve with steamed green vegetables and Roasted Sweet Vegetables (see page 64).

Grated Apple Ice

This is a lovely cooling dessert that can be great for soothing a menopausal hot flush or simply to refresh you when you are feeling low. The combination of the pectin fibre in the apples and the D-limonene in the lemon helps to reduce oestrogen burdens, support the liver generally and relieve constipation, which is a common result of female hormone imbalance.

You should be able to find the rose or orange blossom water at a Middle Eastern grocer or in good supermarkets.

Serves 4

4 Granny Smith apples (or another sharp variety)

juice of 1 lemon

2 tablespoons clear honey

2 tablespoons rose or orange blossom water

4 ice cubes

4 sprigs of fresh mint

1   Peel and grate the apples into a glass bowl, reserving 4 thin slices for the garnish. Squeeze the lemon juice all over the apples to stop them discolouring, and stir well. Add the honey and rose or orange blossom water and stir it all again.

2   Chill for at least 2 hours in the fridge. Before serving, crush the ice cubes in a blender or using a mortar and pestle, and add to the apple mix. Roughly tear the mint leaves and stir into the apple ice. Serve garnished with the slices of apple.

Which lifestyle changes best help balance female hormones?

This advice also applies to male reproductive hormones, as everyone is prey to the damaging effects of modern environmental influences. The more we can be aware of what we are exposing ourselves to within our homes and on our bodies, the more choice we have to buy and use products that support both our own health and that of the planet. Caring for something larger than ourselves is also extremely supportive for health and mood.

Avoid artificial oestrogens

These are common hormone-disrupters found in sources such as cling film/plastic wrap, plastic bottles and non-organic dairy products and meats – where they are used to keep cows lactating and to fatten up livestock. Plastics, petroleum products, tap water and non-organic meat and dairy produce contain xenoestrogens – false oestrogens that disrupt hormone balance – and they should be avoided. Where possible, use stainless-steel and glass containers, don't reuse plastic bottles, buy organic toiletries (that say 'parabens free'), choose organic dairy and meat and definitely do not put more flexible plastics near fats, such as wrapping cheese in cling film/plastic wrap. Oestrogens found in the contraceptive pill and hormone-releasing IUDs can also elevate oestrogen levels.

Avoid toxins and pollutants

Toxins and heavy metals from any source such as cadmium in cigarettes, lead in traffic fumes, tap water, pesticides in non-organic foods and additives are hard for the body to detoxify. They are sometimes 'dumped' in the least life-threatening places in the body, such as the reproductive organs. As well as being toxic to the body, they can rob it of the very antioxidant vitamins and minerals that protect it and that are essential for the detoxification processes. Use wooden or plastic utensils to avoid 'metal on metal' scraping on pans, avoid food in tin cans and mercury-toxic fish such as tuna and swordfish.

Exercise

We are back to where we began with lifestyle – our inherent need to continually move. In context here, exercise and avoiding being sedentary is necessary to help deliver hormones to cells and to support circulation to all organs involved in hormone balance. Yes, this does mean the more obvious and direct reproductive organs, but also the adrenals, liver, thyroid, pancreas and, of course, the brain – all part of the symphony of our bodily functions.

TOP TIPS FOR BALANCING FEMALE HORMONES

In addition to advice from previous chapters:

- Prioritize liver and digestive support for hormone regulation, especially if constipated.
- Have your iron levels tested, if relevant.
- Include phytoestrogens in your diet daily, especially traditional forms of soy.
- Eat 3–4 portions of cruciferous veg daily.
- Experiment with using traditional mushrooms.
- Add in the active form of vitamin B6 (P-5-P) alongside magnesium, if needed.
- Consider the herb appropriate for your needs, consulting a herbalist if possible.
- Include seaweed, sesame seeds, beans and boron-rich foods in your diet.
- Avoid xenoestrogen sources, toxins and pollutants as much as possible, especially soft plastics.
- Avoid a sedentary lifestyle.

CHAPTER 9

FEEL-GOOD DIET BASICS

Now we've explored the various facets that allow us to achieve our best mood, energy, sleep and digestion, it is helpful to have an overview of what this means practically, day to day.

The basics of any healthy, balanced diet are:

- Freshness.
- Variety.
- Eating food as close to its natural state as possible.
- Plenty of fluids and fibre.

These basics translate into practice like this:

- Drink at least 1.5 litres (2½ pints) of pure water or herbal teas throughout the day, between meals.
- Eat fresh, colourful vegetables – raw, lightly steamed or stir-fried, twice a day. About 6–8 portions is optimal, 4–5 minimal.
- Have at least two pieces of fresh fruit daily.
- Eat plenty of fibre-rich foods, such as beans, lentils, whole grains, fruit and vegetables.
- Eat a variety of proteins (including some vegetable protein, even if you are not vegetarian): eggs, organic

meat, sustainable oily and white fish, beans, fermented soy, organic dairy produce – including from goat and sheep, nuts and seeds.

- Eat a variety of foods to ensure that you are getting the full spectrum of required nutrients. Even the healthiest foods, if eaten repeatedly, may leave you short of any nutrients it does not contain.
- Limit the amount of sugar you add to foods and drinks and avoid it in sweetened foods.
- Limit your intake of refined foods (white bread, white rice and so on), processed foods and fast foods.
- Limit your intake of tea and coffee; and replace with herbal, spice and fruit teas.
- Limit your intake of trans fats and fried foods – grill/broil, bake, poach or steam instead.
- Be careful not to overcook food, as heat destroys many valuable nutrients – try to steam or quickly stir-fry vegetables, for example, and enjoy eating them 'crunchy', rather than boiling them until they are completely soft. Whenever possible, eat vegetables raw. The closer a food is to its natural state when you eat it, the more nutrients it will provide.
- Limit your alcohol intake and avoid cigarettes.
- Ensure your food is as free of unhelpful pesticides and additives as possible.

Washing fruit and vegetables

Always wash all your fresh fruits and vegetables thoroughly, even – or perhaps especially – the organic ones. The easiest way to do this is to fill the sink with water, add a few crystals of potassium permanganate (available at any chemist) and a capful of vinegar and put all the fruit and vegetables in to soak. Rinse well. Some, such as leeks and strawberries, are best washed just before you use them, rather than before you store them in the fridge.

Organic

Sadly, eating fresh, unprocessed food will not guarantee that your body gets all the nutrients it needs. The balanced-diet argument is partly based on the notion that our soils are rich in minerals that are absorbed by the plants growing in them, which we subsequently eat. Yet with today's intensive farming methods and artificial fertilizers, plants no longer need naturally mineral-rich soil to grow into the bumper-crop, over-sized, uniform fruits and vegetables we now expect to see on our supermarket shelves.

Also, we do not always eat fruit and vegetables in season, many have been picked before they are ripe, stored for long periods of time then shipped across the world, none of which does their nutrient content much good. Frozen foods are often richer in nutrients than some fresh because they are picked at their optimum ripeness and immediately preserved by the freezing process. Ideally, your balanced diet should consist of as many organic foods as possible, bought fresh from producers who do not use chemicals.

Buy as much organic produce as you can afford and is available. That way you minimize your toxin intake, are supporting a more sustainable environment and helping bring down the cost of organic food. Don't be fooled into thinking that if something is organic it is, de facto, good for you. An organic biscuit and an organic coffee made with organic cream and sugar, is still high in sugar, wheat, caffeine and saturated fat.

Eating out

Eating away from home – whether during the working day, at business lunches or going out for dinner – is increasingly common. It may seem like hard work to follow the principles of good mood food when you do not have absolute control

THE COMPONENTS OF A HEALTHY MEAL

This diagram represents the proportions of fresh vegetables, protein and (non-gluten) starch in an ideal meal for keeping blood sugar levels as even as possible. While such a meal is being digested and its nutrients are released to produce energy, dramatic fluctuations in blood sugar levels are avoided.

Sticking to these proportions of fresh vegetables, protein and starch most of the time will help you to maintain even moods and energy levels. However, bear in mind that the diagram need not be applied to every meal you eat. For example, some people (especially with blood sugar balance issues) fare much better by replacing the starchy carb part with more vegetables or nuts and seeds. Also, a breakfast meal of full-fat yoghurt with berries will differ wildly from this diagram. So we suggest using this diagram as a basic eating guide for applicable meals; at its simplest level, it shows how at least half of our diet needs to be vegetables for optimal wellness!

Also within this plate can be included roughly:

- 10 per cent healthy fats.
- 5 per cent concentrated nutrients – as herbs and spices.

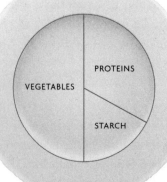

over your meals, but with only a little bit of planning it can actually be very easy to do.

For example, breakfast at work or on the run could be a piece of fruit, a small pot of plain yoghurt and a handful of nuts or seeds. A good take-away lunch might be a baked potato with a protein-rich filling (such as salmon, cheese or eggs) and a salad; sushi; rice salad; soup (keep your own rice, oat or rye crackers at your desk to have with it); or a bag of raw, washed vegetables from the supermarket with cooked chicken, goat's cheese or houmous.

If you are going out for a meal, my advice would be to just enjoy it: choose whatever you fancy from the menu and make the most of the occasion. However, if you want to follow the recommendations in this book strictly, or you have to eat out regularly, here are some suggestions to bear in mind when selecting your meal:

- Choose a light starter, such as rocket/arugula salad, grilled/broiled vegetables or a non-creamy soup.
- Go for a simple main course or ask for it to be cooked plainly, for example, griddled sea bass or baked chicken without a rich sauce.
- Order plenty of fresh, lightly cooked vegetables or a large salad to go with your main dish, and explain that you would like to have more of these vegetables than potatoes or rice.
- If you order a dessert, share it with someone or just choose a fruit salad.
- Order a peppermint tea instead of coffee – this will not only help your digestion but also refresh your palate.
- If you are drinking alcohol, always have it with food and start with a large glass of mineral water, then alternate drinking a glass of wine with a glass of water, or drink spritzers (white wine with soda water).

YOUR framework for a GOOD MOOD

With these basic guidelines you can use the recipes in this book to explore and address your particular mood issues or needs. The advice in Chapter 1 lays out the framework for a mood-supporting nutritional day that sets you up for blood sugar balance, the keystone of sustained brain function, response, focus and energy. As all of the recipes in this book support this foundation in some way, here they all are laid out in the categories we use to describe meals, but remember that you do not need to be confined by these labels; a soup, stew or salad works really well for breakfast and many of the breakfast meals make great light suppers or snacks.

This is about finding your rhythm, paying attention to your mind-body responses and trusting what you discover as you experiment with new tastes and ideas. Write down any observations, personal variations and how these worked for you in a dedicated notebook or document, then you have a guide to come back to whenever you wander into less-helpful habits. You can also make notes and bookmarks within these pages when you find a passage that really speaks to you. The more you can understand why something works for you, the more likely you are to keep it up.

A 7-day good mood plan

Using these recipes, it can be helpful to create a set plan for yourself to provide a framework to follow as you experiment with changing your diet. This can free you to simply focus on how the suggestions make you feel and be with the emotions and responses that arise, as well as the physical symptoms.

Seven days might look like the table opposite, but it is a good idea to make a similar table (for one, two or more weeks) and sit down to consider your own plan according to the time you have to prepare food each day, personal limitations such

Breakfast	Lunch	Dinner
Scrambled Eggs on Rye	Protein (fish, eggs, meat, beans, tofu, nuts, goat's cheese) with Bitters and Artichoke Salad	Thai-style Noodle Soup
Very Berry Smoothie	Seatown Kedgeree	Protein (fish, eggs, meat, beans, tofu, nuts, goat's cheese) with Proper Green Salad
Buckwheat Crepes	Chicken or Tofu Sesame Stir-Fry	Quinoa with Roasted Vegetables
Apple Porridge	Protein (fish, eggs, meat, beans, tofu, nuts, goat's cheese) with Red Cabbage and Feta Salad	Mushroom Pâté with crackers and salad
Poached Eggs with Asparagus	Baby Spinach and Goat's Cheese Salad	Chunky Vegetable Soup
Omega-rich Bircher Muesli	Protein (fish, eggs, meat, beans, tofu, nuts, goat's cheese) with Tabouleh	Miso and Seaweed Broth with Tempeh
Frittata	Trout with Sunflower Seeds and Roasted Vegetable Salad	Lentils with Spinach

as a family to cook for or a long commute, likes and dislikes, ethical choices and extra needs for vegans, what has worked for you before and what level of change you feel you can handle at this time. Your choices need to feel achievable and practical; you do not need to simply change everything at once if you think the suggestions are a long way away from your current eating habits. It is better to make a few simple changes and feel the benefits so that you are motivated to continue and keep them up. Then they make sense to you and you will remember why you are doing them; this is the route to long-term change.

You can also set a specific time for a plan where you follow the suggestions as a more dedicated period of mood 'detox'. If you are going down this route, make sure you follow all of the lifestyle suggestions, including plenty of relaxation and recovery time, as you may feel a little worse or need to allow deep sleep (or fatigue) to heal you. Also make sure you are well hydrated (see pages 146–7), that you exercise and have periods of active relaxation (see pages 131–2) to allow optimal change and feel the benefits

You might also want to add in some specific tweaks for your individual needs, for example:

- A snack mid-afternoon to pre-empt a blood sugar dip or to see you through until dinner (see page 38–39).
- A snack before bed if waking in the night has been an issue (see page 213).
- A bigger or extra-starchy carbohydrate portion (see suggestions on page 186) at lunch if you feel hungry mid-afternoon, are exercising a lot or experiencing cravings later – play around with this to see what best sustains you. You can add in for dinner, too, but you'll find you do get used to less food at night (it encourages hunger for breakfast) and that will support any weight-management efforts.
- Reducing sugar before you reduce caffeine (see page 52).
- A daily prescribed treat of 40 g (1½ oz) plain chocolate (see page 69).
- If you tend to have big sugar cravings, or overeat or bing, pay particular attention to the advice in Chapter 6 on Appetite Regulation and try eating baked potatoes for lunch.
- Reduce high alcohol intake slowly (see page 178).

It can be useful to enlist the help of technology here. Online shopping can be great for saving the ingredient items you often buy to make your favourite recipes. It can take a little time to set up, but once you have a 'favourites' shopping list, most online supermarkets will also let you make a list that you can easily come back to and use to order again. So if there is a time where you need help getting back on track, you can return back to your plan and simply repeat your order for easy delivery.

Reflective practice

You will gain most insight on your own personal needs from what you experience with each meal and food variation if you reflect on how they made you feel and note what worked for you, what didn't and even where you were confused or may have more questions. Journalling or making notes helps this process and links the sensory experience of eating with memory and future decision-making.

You can ask yourself these questions, or any similar that help you make a 'map' of what your body and mind respond to positively – and what they do not!

- How did I feel when I sat down, paid attention and chewed my food thoroughly?
- How do particular tastes register in my body and my brain?
- Which textures make me feel most satisfied?
- In which emotional states do I enjoy my food the most?
- Which foods do I use for self-medication, soothing and numbing?
- How do I feel if I make a choice to soothe my brain if I feel agitated?
- How do I feel if I eat something helpful for mood and then wait to notice the responses (beyond the immediate) in my body-mind?
- What are the subtle and larger positive changes?
- How is it difficult or challenging to keep these up?
- Which foods work best for me to be able to stay on course with the changes I want to make?
- Which lifestyle factors are most useful for my relationship with food?

Even if such self-enquiry seems strange and new, you'll soon get used to directing your attention inwards towards your sensory experience and the ripples that creates. The more we can foster such awareness, the more choice we have in our responses and the less inclined we are to knee-jerk reactions to stress and emotional distress. This is how we can help reduce cravings and instead be with any difficult feelings they provoke; being kind to yourself and practising self-compassion means not needing to judge if it doesn't always go according to plan – we are all human, after all!

A 14-day cleanse

The changes above and outlined throughout the book will support your detoxification processes in a progressive way that allows you to function and relate to change. Once you've introduced these and found your rhythm you may feel a more dedicated period of cleanse would be helpful, particularly if you have some habits that feel a bit 'stuck' and you would like to address them, let go of them and move forward.

Essentially this is eating within the framework outlined in the 7-day plan, but going a little further to reduce sugar, caffeine and other burdens on your gut and liver. This means that the foods you eat during these 14 days won't be so different from those that suit you day to day, and it's not that you are doing a 'specific regime' but rather learning to eat in a new and sustainable way and understanding that sometimes we need periods where we are more 'clean', to reset our choices and taste habits. The more you do this, the easier it becomes to eat in the way that makes you feel best, most of the time – and you don't beat yourself up when you don't!

This 14-day programme is designed to:

- Fuel the body optimally.
- Kick-start new habits.
- Cleanse all your body systems.
- Enhance body system function.
- Restore control and balance to your body and moods.

After following such a programme, most people find they feel physically energized, and mentally and emotionally reinvigorated. However, if you are ill or on medication, you should not embark on this programme without first asking your doctor or nutritionist for advice.

Getting ready to cleanse

Gradually start reducing your intake of tea, coffee, alcohol and sugar, so that you do not have to go 'cold turkey' on day one. For some people, such changes are very dramatic to their normal routine, so you may want to introduce them slowly over a couple of weeks before launching fully into the cleansing programme, following the advice in Chapter 1. This way, you are being more gentle on your system and you will be less likely to feel unwell as you detox. Make sure you stock up on all the foodstuffs you will need for the programme.

Your food on the programme

Once you begin the 14-day programme, your daily food intake (organic as far as possible) should include:

- At least 1½ litres (2½ pints) of non-sugary or caffeinated fluids between meals – although this may take some getting used to, it is quite easy to achieve if you start the day with a glass of hot water with a squeeze of lemon or grated ginger root, then have a herbal tea or water between meals.

- Three pieces of fresh fruit – vary the fruit you have, and choose those that are in season and, ideally, locally grown, as these are likely to be fresher. Berries are the best choice for blood sugar support and limit more sugary varieties such as bananas and grapes.
- Fresh vegetables at lunch and dinner (even breakfast, too) – have a variety and choose different colours.
- Fresh vegetable and fruit juices – for a particularly cleansing juice add some greens, such as spinach, broccoli or kale, and some fresh ginger. Carrot, apple, celery, grapefruit, kale and ginger juice is particularly delicious. Add a dessertspoon of flax oil or soaked flaxseeds (see page 114) to slow down the sugar release of the vegetables and fruit with their fibre removed.
- Plenty of naturally fibre-rich foods, such as beans, lentils, whole grains and root vegetables (see cooking advice for beans on pages 59 and 156).
- For protein, have fermented soy products (such as tofu and tempeh), beans, lentils, an egg, piece of fish and the odd piece of meat as needed for energy.
- For any starchy foods, have brown basmati rice, baked sweet potatoes, buckwheat pasta or noodles, quinoa, buckwheat, rice cakes, oat cakes – or a green veg such as broccoli, asparagus and cabbage.

To give your digestive system and detoxification pathways a rest, avoid or cut down on the following:

- Alcohol – avoid completely for this time.
- Coffee, tea – have herbal, fruit and spice teas instead.
- Fried or fatty foods, including chips, crisps, bacon and cured meats.
- Dairy products – for example, cheese, yoghurt, cream, butter, ice cream, fromage frais – with the exception of

organic, live plain yoghurt and organic butter, although you can use tahini (sesame spread) instead; use coconut, almond or hemp milk and coconut yoghurt.

- Any foods containing artificial additives or sweeteners.
- Processed and refined foods, including 'ready meals'.
- Sugary foods and drinks – have an occasional fruit bar or a little fruit or dried fruit instead.
- Wheat – bread, pasta, crackers, biscuits, muffins, wheat cereals, couscous, ordinary noodles (including egg noodles), cakes, bagels. Many people who have a food sensitivity (see pages 179-81) or at least find it difficult to digest discover that they feel less bloated and lethargic when they cut down on wheat, especially bread.
- Limit your intake of other gluten grains – that is oats, rye and barley – to once every two days. These can be avoided and replaced with loads of vegetables for more weight loss and digestive relief.

To support your diet, also:

- Put 2 dessertspoons of organic, golden flaxseeds (available in healthfood stores, avoid the brown variety) in a glass of water overnight then chew and drink the mixture in the morning. Flaxseeds are cleansing and also help bulk out your food as it passes through the digestive tract.
- Take a liver 'flush' first thing each morning: mix the juice of 1 grapefruit and 1 lemon, 2 tablespoons of extra-virgin olive oil, 1 crushed clove garlic and a 2½ cm (1 inch) piece of fresh root ginger (grated).
- Buy a firm-bristle brush from a healthfood shop or chemist and brush your skin daily before you shower. This enhances lymphatic flow, which improves waste-disposal mechanisms. Brush in steady upward movements towards the heart.

- Take some exercise daily or at least every other day. This can be walking, swimming, cycling, yoga or whatever form of exercise you prefer. It is best to avoid particularly vigorous kinds of exercise as they can be too much for the detoxing body.
- Include 'active relaxation' (see pages 131–2).
- Make sure you are getting adequate sleep (at least seven hours a night) so that your body has time to rest and regenerate.

Supplements in a nutshell

Here is a roundup of the supplement advice throughout the book, with a basic multivitamin and mineral plus vitamin C as abase and then references to others mentioned in various chapters. This advice is useful to support the changes described in the plan and programme above. You can buy these supplements at healthfood shops or online, or ask your nutritionist or herbalist to recommend good brands.

Multivitamin and -mineral –to include: B vitamins Chromium 400mcg Zinc 5–15mg	Pay for quality or you won't receive the right amount of nutrients in an absorbable form.	Advised to meet the shortfall of nutrients in the modern diet, due to stress, poor soil quality and distribution methods. Energy nutrients to support blood sugar balance. Also shown to support weight-loss efforts.
Vitamin C 1,000mg a day Avoid cheap, effervescent types with sweeteners added	**High amounts** strawberries, spring greens, blackcurrants, red peppers, watercress, oranges, lemons, kiwi fruit **Moderate amounts** grapefruit, nectarines, banana, spring onion/ scallion, parsley, tomatoes, peaches, raspberries	Poor levels in modern food. Higher need for this nutrient if under stress or exposed to pollution. Naturally anti-inflammatory. May help reduce cravings. Supports liver detoxification.

Plus possible:

- Magnesium - see page 54–5
- L-Theanine - see page 56
- Omega 3 oil or vegan algae form - see page 112
- Antioxidant complex - see page 117
- Probiotic - see page 149
- Aloe vera - see page 150
- Milk thistle - see page 150
- Digestive enzymes - see page 150
- Liver support - see page 150
- Sleep support - see pages 214–15
- Vitamin D3 - see pages 118–9
- Iron - see page 243

Feel-good strategies

Although this book focuses primarily on the nutritional aspects of improving mood, many other forms of therapy can make a significant difference to how you feel. Looking after your body and mind should be a holistic experience that encompasses all aspects of what it is to be human.

Getting it all moving

One way of looking at low moods and fatigue is as stagnation and rigid patterns in your body and mind dragging you down. If you exercise, you are starting to create movement, fluidity and change. Any lifestyle aimed at getting or maintaining a healthy body and mind must involve some sort of regular physical activity and a recognition that exercise is inherent in raising mood. It is something all of us are aware of; some of us do it without fail, some of us get round to it intermittently (and then remember how great it feels) and some of us ignore it completely. Unless you are in the first category and therefore need no encouragement at all, the key to incorporating regular exercise into your weekly routine is to choose a form of physical activity that stimulates you, one that you enjoy and one that is appropriate for your level of strength and fitness.

Exercise promotes the release of mood-improving chemicals – such as endorphins, noradrenaline (linked to drive and motivation), dopamine and serotonin. These chemicals not only give you a boost during your actual workout, but for some time afterwards as well.

The first step in beginning an exercise programme is the all-important decision to get moving. Once you have started this journey, it can create the motivation to keep going and feel the changes to mood, appetite, cravings and health that this can bring. As exercise is so important to help instigate and keep up nutritional change, here are some tips:

- Check with your doctor first if you have any doubt about your ability to exercise, for example, if you have reason to be worried about your cardiac health or you suffer from any bone or muscle problems.
- Always start gently and build up slowly. If you are exercising at a club or in a class, talk to your trainer or teacher about what is best for you.
- Exercise at the time of day that feels right for you – there's no point in dragging yourself out of bed 90 minutes earlier than usual if it is just going to make you feel more exhausted and miserable. For many people, exercising towards the end of the day (but not too late in the evening) is best.
- Exercising before a meal can help metabolism and how you digest food.
- Ideally, after eating, you should wait for two hours before exercising.

- Even if it is hard to get yourself going, it is important that you actually want to exercise, so choose an activity that inspires you and surround it with motivating add-ons, such as music and wearing comfortable, appropriate clothing/shoes.
- Exercising with a friend can help to motivate you.
- Exercise need not be fancy and expensive and require special gear. Walking is our most natural and necessary form of exercise: you can do it anywhere and it's free. Walking for just 20 minutes a day can make a difference. You could even incorporate it into your journey to work, your lunch break or going to pick up the children from school. Make sure you walk in a safe area that is well-lit if you walk at night and get out into greenery to lower stress hormones as often as you can.
- Mindful and meditative movement forms such as yoga, t'ai chi and qigong also encourage awareness and a positive relationship with your body.

Talking therapies

Because low moods are very often precipitated by low self-esteem, a traumatic event, chronic stress in domestic or working life, repeated destructive behavioural patterns or internalized anger, talking therapies are usually very helpful to break such patterns, to learn to deal with certain situations or to learn to accept oneself. After all, life is always going to present us with difficulties, and it is how we perceive these and how we handle them that makes the difference. Counselling or some sort of psychotherapy can be extremely useful. If you embark on such a programme, bear in mind that therapy does not offer a 'cure', is not always easy and often involves a long-term investment of time and effort. However, your therapist can lend a non-judgemental, listening ear along the journey and the rewards, in terms of your emotional wellbeing, can be considerable.

Exploring acceptance, self-worth and how one deals with life events can be invaluable in overcoming persistent or recurring low moods or depression. It is often our unconscious reactions to stressful or emotionally challenging events that keeps us coming back to these patterns. We also need to practise mindfulness and embodied awareness (see page 199) alongside to instill a grounded sense of safety in the body and not simply talk to the mind.

There are countless types of psychotherapy to choose from, but it appears that it is not the particular school of training that makes the most difference, but the strength of the bond between the therapist and client.

LIFE COACHING

If the thought of entering into a therapy programme of any sort does not appeal, perhaps life coaching would be more appropriate for you. Working with a life coach can give you the confidence and ability to move forward in the areas of your life where you feel you are in a rut, especially if work stress, workaholism or the tricky boundaries of self-employment are involved. Life coaches recognize that it is often our own high expectations, married with frustrations and a sense of stagnation, that can leave us feeling low. A professional life coach, who can often provide sessions by telephone or email, can help you in a variety of ways. He or she may:

- Show you how to set more appropriate, realistic goals and then reach them.
- Encourage you to achieve more by working on ways to take down the barriers to doing so.
- Help you to focus better, to produce results more efficiently.
- Provide you with the tools, support and structure to improve any area of your life.

Alternative approaches

For many of us with busy lifestyles, making time for ourselves is surprisingly difficult, and it is often something we relegate to the bottom of our list of priorities. However, 'me time' is crucial to balancing everything else that is going on in our lives.

When you are feeling down, there are countless simple ways that you can give yourself a boost. Just taking some time out from your daily routine to relax and rejuvenate your body and mind – whether that is in the form of having a bath, playing with the children or doing some exercise – can make a tremendous difference.

If you have been feeling persistently low for a long time, in addition to adopting the nutritional strategies described in this book, you may also want to try a complementary therapy that addresses stress-related problems and helps you to rediscover harmony between your body and mind.

Acupuncture

This is the ancient Eastern art of using very fine needles, which are painlessly inserted into special points along meridians (energy lines) in the body, to gently correct imbalances in the body's natural energy flow. A very powerful treatment, acupuncture can help deal with both physical and mental conditions, and has great results with stress-related conditions. Scientific trials have found acupuncture to be at least as effective as drug therapy in combating depression.

Homoeopathy

This is one of the truly holistic therapies that, although seemingly incredibly subtle, can have remarkable effects. You are given a specifically chosen remedy by your homoeopath – in an infinitesimal dosage – which stimulates the body to heal any imbalances.

Herbal medicine

Both the traditional Chinese and Western use of plants for medical purposes are almost as old as humankind itself. In the West, the best-known herb for helping balance mood is St John's Wort, which is among the most widely prescribed antidepressants in Germany. It is believed to work by increasing the levels of serotonin in circulation in the body. It is best to visit a qualified medical herbalist who can give you a prescription of this, or other herbs tailored to your personal needs.

Flower essences

These essences (such as Australian Bush Flower Essences or Bach Flower Remedies) are another very subtle but effective way of addressing emotional imbalances. You can buy them at most health shops and chemists, and there are several books and websites available that can help you choose which essences would be most appropriate for you. They can also be taken under the guidance of an experienced health practitioner.

Aromatherapy

The concentrated essential oils of plants are used for massage, inhalation, compresses, baths and in special burners. When chosen by a trained aromatherapist, the blend of oils used can help to relieve a range of both emotional and physical conditions.

Massage

There are many types of massage available – including myofascial release, aromatherapy, deep tissue and shiatsu. The best way to find out which is suited to you is to contact a local natural health clinic and discuss your wants and needs. When performed by a skilled practitioner, massage can have very profound physical and emotional effects.

GLOSSARY

Acetylcholine
The main neurotransmitter for communication between brain neurons that are responsible for, among other things, memory and cognitive thinking.

Adrenaline
Also known as epinephrine, this hormone is secreted by the adrenal glands as part of the body's response to stress. Adrenaline plays a role in effecting physiological changes that include faster breathing, raised heart rate and increased levels of blood glucose, all of which are intended to enable the body to respond effectively to a stressful situation.

Amino acid
A building block of protein. All the proteins in the body are made up of combinations of any number of amino acids, of which there are about twenty in total.

Antioxidant
A substance – nutrient or enzyme – which can 'disarm' an oxidant. In other words, antioxidants neutralize the potentially damaging effects of oxidation. Key antioxidant nutrients are vitamins A, C and E. Fresh fruit and vegetables, nuts, seeds and whole grains are all particularly rich sources of antioxidants.

Carbohydrate

A sugar or starch that is used by the body primarily as fuel for energy production. Rice, pasta, bread, potatoes and sugar are rich sources of carbohydrates.

Cortisol

A hormone secreted by the adrenal glands in response to stress. Cortisol plays a part in effecting the physiological changes that help the body deal with the stress, perceived or real. One of cortisol's key roles is to increase the supply of glucose to the brain and other tissues. Cortisol helps reduce inflammation, but also appears to interfere with the levels of the mood-boosting neurotransmitters serotonin and dopamine that the body produces.

DHA

DHA, or docosahexaenoic acid, is an essential fatty acid which is found in fish, and can also be produced in the body from fats contained in flaxseeds, hemp seeds and walnuts. DHA is used in the body in the lining of nerves and cell membranes.

Dopamine

Like serotonin, dopamine is a neurotransmitter involved in mood and motivation. Dopamine can be made in the body from the amino acids phenylalanine and tyrosine. EPA, or eicosapentaenoic acid, is an essential fatty acid that is in the same 'family' as DHA.

EPA

EPA is found in fish, and can also be made in the body from fats contained in flaxseeds, hemp seeds and walnuts. EPA has many uses in the body, including forming part of the lining of nerves and cell membranes.

Essential fatty acids (EFAs)

A group of fats (oils) essential for many vital functions in the body, including healthy brain and nerve cells, balanced hormones, energy production and well-hydrated skin. EFAs can only be obtained from the diet; rich sources are nuts, seeds and oily fish.

Glucose

A type of sugar which is the prime source of fuel for energy in the brain as well as the rest of the body. The body converts carbohydrates into sugars such as glucose during the digestive process.

Gluten

A protein found in grains such as wheat, oats, rye and barley.

Glycaemic index (GI)

A scale that measures the rate at which a particular food is digested and released as glucose into the bloodstream. The faster a food raises blood-sugar levels, the higher it is rated on the GI scale.

Neuron

A nerve cell, sometimes called a neurone. Nerve cells exist throughout the body and brain.

Neurotransmitter

A chemical in the body that facilitates the transmission of impulses (messages) through the nervous system, from one neuron to the next.

Nutrients

All chemical reactions that take place in the body depend on a regular supply of 'micro' nutrients, such as vitamins and minerals, and 'macro' nutrients, including protein, carbohydrates, fats and water.

Oxidants

Molecules that are byproducts of oxygen and can be likened to 'sparks' from anything that burns, including cigarettes and food, as well as the combustion of glucose in our cells to make energy. Oxidants can damage cells, thereby accelerating ageing and causing disease. Antioxidants help counter such damage.

Phosphatidylcholine (PC)

A type of phospholipid containing choline, which is incorporated into healthy cell membranes and needed to make acetylcholine. PC is also contained in bile where it contributes to the proper digestion of fats. Lecithin (found in soy, eggs and as a food supplement) is a source of PC.

Phospholipid

A substance made of phosphorus and lipids (fats), phospholipids form an important part of human cell membranes, including those of neurons.

Probiotics

A term used to describe the beneficial 'bacteria' in our gut, such as Lactobacillus acidophilus and bifidobacteria, that are needed for healthy digestion. Probiotics are available as food supplements and are also found in live plain yoghurt.

Protein
Made of amino acids, proteins are used in the body to form the main structures, including all cells, as well as enzymes, hormones and neurotransmitters. Fish, poultry, meat, milk, yoghurt, cheese and beans such as soy are rich sources of protein.

Saturated fat
A type of fat found mainly in animal-derived foods such as meat and dairy products. Saturated fats are not essential for human health and should not be consumed in large quantities.

Serotonin
A mood-boosting neurotransmitter that is involved in numerous processes in the body, including sending out the signals that control appetite. Serotonin is derived from the amino acid tryptophan.

Trans fatty acid
A type of fat that has been transformed by exposure to excess heat or light, changing its chemical structure and rendering it harmful to the body. EFAs are particularly susceptible to oxidation damage, which can turn them into trans fatty acids. Many commercially produced oils contain trans fatty acids.

Tryptophan
An amino acid which is particularly abundant in bananas, chicken, figs, milk, seaweeds, sunflower seeds, tuna, turkey and yoghurt. Tryptophan can be converted in the body into the neurotransmitter serotonin.

Unsaturated fat

Considered to be far more healthy than saturated fats, unsaturated fats are found in vegetable sources, including oils such as olive, sunflower, safflower, rapeseed, soy, peanut and sesame. Unsaturated fats can be further sub-divided into monounsaturated and polyunsaturated fats (the latter is another name for essential fatty acids).

INDEX

Recipe page references are in **bold.**